The International Library of Psychology

INVENTION AND UNCONSCIOUS

Founded by C. K. Ogden

The International Library of Psychology

COGNITIVE PSYCHOLOGY
In 21 Volumes

PREFACE

" I would, therefore, strongly advise the reader to use man, and the present races of man, and the growing inventions and conceptions of man, as his guide, if he would seek to form an independent judgment on the development of organic life. For all growth is only somebody making something "—S. BUTLER : *Life and Habit.*

IN this book, M. Montmasson is concerned to demonstrate a fact of the first importance, easily overlooked. The fact is this, that human inventions in the widest sense of the word, are products of the unconscious. Now this thesis is one already commonly accepted, in a vague way, by all but a few metaphysicians. But its exact implications have been hardly thought out. For instance, it is incompatible with the equally common assumption that the creative genius exhibits mind at a stage of evolution beyond that of its otherwise highest point—human self-consciousness.[1] On the contrary, creative activity of a highly ingenious description is exhibited by organisms very low in the scale of being ; while at the other end of the scale, the typical powerful and controlling human " master-mind ", capable of a range and content of conscious grasp far beyond that of common humanity, is normally entirely uncreative. Its power lies in its complete consciousness of every element in a given situation, and of all the known and tried methods of meeting situations. The *creation* of new methods can almost always be traced to individuals of quite another type—one often deserving the epithet " impossible ".

M. Montmasson's treatment of the subject is entirely from the point of view of introspective psychology, and the Editor therefore suggested that a few pages devoted to indicating the connections with other systems

[1] E.g in *Nature*, 8th March, 1930, " . . . if, as one seems justified in assuming, invention is one of the highest forms of thought."

of psychology and biology might be of value to the reader.

Human invention, even in the widest sense of the word, is not a phenomenon of nature to be placed in a class by itself. The productions of inventive genius serve two ends : utility and pleasure. In either case they take the form, as a rule, of instructions to the rest of mankind as to how either a useful adaptation to or of an environment may be effected, or how subjectively pleasureable feelings may be obtained. But it is commonplace that the most ingenious adaptations for use and, frequently also, pleasure, occur in all organisms down to the lowest ; and that nowhere in organic nature can a line be drawn which definitely separates adaptations of the nature of our own inventions from the adaptations which result in new species.

We are thus driven to the conclusion that *human invention is the psychical counterpart of the modifications of structure, instinct, and habit by which living species have been produced.*

There is to-day in psychology an active element which seeks to advance by collating what we know of mind by introspection, psychoanalysis, and other similar methods, with our purely objective observation of the behaviour of living matter. Thus Dr. W. M. Marston, for instance, in seeking to investigate human emotion assumed that its primary elements must correspond to the possible types of response of living matter to stimulus. A body organism such as an amœba may react to external stimulus in several (Marston names four) fundamental ways. He assumes that we, too, can only react in these ways, either singly or combined, and that our subjective sensations, accompanying our response to stimulus, must therefore be also analysable into four fundamental types, or emotional elements. In his hands, this line of research has already borne considerable fruit.

This standpoint bears a certain relationship to vitalism.

The mechanist regards all concern with psychical phenomena in biology as waste of time ; for him, mind is a by-product of the physico-chemical processes which *are* life. Even if this were the case, it is not at all impossible that an examination and analysis of mental processes might serve as a guide in the investigation of the stupendous complexity with which bio-chemistry and bio-physics are confronted. The vitalist, on the other hand, regards the psychical element as essential and, indeed, directive. He has been driven, it is true, from every position which he has taken up on matters of fact, from the time of Wöhler's Urea synthesis onwards. On the other hand, the mechanist has also suffered defeat, though not of a sort leading to the enthronement of his rival. Natural selection as stated by Darwin, and the spontaneous generation of life by the chance formation from its chemical elements of a simple organism, are but two examples of mechanistic assumptions which are regarded to-day almost universally, as refuted by experiment and observation.

The problem of the origin of species, and the transmission by heredity of their characteristics, continues to be the central problem of biology. If human invention can be shown to be its psychical counterpart, a study of it should assist in elucidating the biological question.

At first sight, it would appear possible to draw a rigid line between, say, the sword of a sword-fish and the human lethal weapon of the same name. In the one case, we have undoubtedly the sword present in the animal potentially as a peculiar structure of one or more of its genes, while in the other case, the sword is made by a workman, who has received verbal and practical tradition which goes back to the individual human beings in whose minds all the various peculiarities of the particular sword originated. It is probable that the human invention was made quite independently of any observation of a sword-fish, and it would appear at first sight entirely useless from a serious scientific point of view to stress even so striking an analogy. The sword of the sword-fish is the result of a mutation or a series of mutations, resulting in an admirable adaptation of bodily structure. The sword of man is, it is usually supposed, the result of "thinking" out how best to slay his enemy, of trying out various methods, and of gradually improving his product by the use of suitable methods and materials. In other words, the process by which it originated is supposed to be entirely different; and an analogy between the two kinds of sword is regarded as of no more relevancy than an analogy between the floral designs on a frozen window pane and real flowers.

If it can be shown (a) that human inventions are not the product of this transparent conscious "thinking out"; (b) that at no point can a line be drawn between them and organic adaptations, (c) that they arise in a manner strikingly analogous to the adaptations of organisms; then we shall be obliged to admit that there is in fact more in the analogy than mere superficial similarity.

The first point is dealt with by M. Montmasson. *Inventions are not thought-out.* Thinking-out is a process of envisaging consciously on the one hand all the elements and conditions of a given problematical situation, and on the other hand, all the known and tried, or even suggested means of dealing with it. *New* means and *new* forms are generated in the Unconscious, and furthermore, in that of rare individuals and not of the great majority.

The second point is one for biology. Alongside the infinity of ingenious structural patterns of survival value in lower organisms, we find an equal number of entirely fixed, inborn behaviour patterns, or instincts. No biologist would dream of assigning the latter any other origin, than a modification of the genes. Certain animals, e.g. camels, have special bodily characteristics which permit the storage of food against a time of scarcity. Certain other animals instinctively bury food for the same reason. The latter animals (e.g. squirrels) will go through all the motions of burying food upon a smooth concrete floor. There can be no doubt that these instincts are transmitted in the genes, just as are bodily characteristics for food storage, and that they have arisen by mutation. The old argument used to be that in man " reason " replaced instinct. This argument has received a sufficient battering of recent times, to a point which guidance by reason is totally denied. In reality, we find all the elements of the human type of behaviour in animals. There is a gradual transition from behaviour of the " blind " instinctive type such as that of the squirrel referred to, to behaviour which consists in the application of learned methods to suitable situations. The vogue of the limited behaviourist outlook, applied also to man, is passing ; but it in no way bears upon our argument. An animal or man " conditioned " by its parents or the tribe acts in a way which is entirely similar to that of the " blind " instinct. There is indeed a gradual transition from one to the other. Certain birds are taught by their parents to fly, others fly without any such instruction. It is obvious, of course, that whether what is transmitted by the genes is the " blind " instinct itself, or an equally blind instinct to teach certain habits to the young, the whole affair consists in the transmission from generation to generation of highly " ingenious " and elaborate devices which are useful or pleasureable.

Human everyday reason is, in reality, no more than the power of accurately grasping in consciousness the essentials of a given situation, of recollecting suitable learned means for dealing with such situations. The devising of new means is no part of it ; these as M. Montmasson shows, originate in the unconscious of certain individuals, and are then made part of the common stock of expedients.

The truth of this view is seen by a consideration of

the broad general facts of the adaptation of organisms to their environment. We believe that all the infinitely various living beings have evolved by descent with modification. The old mechanical view is abandoned; we believe that all living creatures sometimes exhibit the faculty of modifying their structure and habits, probably quite rapidly, in such a way as to further their racial survival. This faculty has been exercised innumerable times, and in a manner which we cannot but call ingenious, inventive, and often also artistic, in the highest degree. But the really astonishing thing is the fact that comparatively speaking, it has been exercised but rarely. Its exercise is the exception, not the rule. The rule is that when a species is met by new and adverse conditions it perishes. Normally each species, having originated some quite extraordinary bodily modifications, instincts, or habits, sticks tenaciously and quite conservatively to these even in the face of changed conditions, which may make them disadvantageous.

Precisely the same thing is true of human inventions. Not a tribe of savages exists but has a number of peculiar and highly ingenious contrivances for locomotion; warfare, transport, amusement, obtaining and preparing food, shelter, and clothing. All these contrivances must have originated at some time. Most such tribes live or have lived under conditions of perpetual danger from other savages, wild animals, or nature; and very many of them, as experience shows, possess a brain capacity fully on a level with the average white civilized man. A very little ingenuity would have sufficed to give any one of them a full measure of security against their enemies, human and natural. So far from such invention having been exercised, we find that ingenious and useful contrivances used by one tribe frequently fail to be copied by others in contact with it.

At the same time, no engineer can feel anything but wonder and admiration when examining these primitive inventions. Some of them are marvels of design, of the use of certain materials, chemicals, and natural processes. The conclusion is irresistible that the brain of primitive man, indistinguishable from our own anatomically, was also, on occasion, the equal of our own in creative ingenuity. The artist, and especially the modern artist, is equally ready to concede equality in his own sphere of creation.

What actually happens is seen, in its most recent and grandest phase, in the rise and development of civilizations. In a certain area, among a primitive population with a past history of long comparative stability, a powerful impulse makes itself felt. In the wide sense of the word invention, an epoch of inventive activity sets in. In religion, government, art, science, literature, philosophy, creation proceeds rapidly ; history is made from one generation to the next, even from one decade to the next.

This process is one with which we are familiar, for we live in such an epoch. Creative activity is at its height. Comparatively few in number though they be compared to the 300,000,000 individuals who are concerned in the progress of Western European civilization, the fertile, original minds are vast in number. For some thousands of years or so, they have poured forth ideas, first in religion, philosophy, theology, architecture, then government, painting, music, science, then science and technology. These ideas have been eagerly seized upon and developed ; each generation has lived, thought, worked, played, and fought differently from its predecessor or its successor. Not altogether gladly, as we know. The conservative tendency, though no longer triumphant, has acted as a powerful brake.

In all other civilizations, apparently, it has triumphed in the end, or else the creative spirit has exhausted itself. Advance ceases, a grandiose and immensely complicated structure continues almost unchanged from generation to generation ; as did the original primitive tribal life out of which it grew. And in spite of its impressive intellectuality, in spite of the numbers of "first-class brains" which it will be found to contain, it almost always fails completely to meet changed conditions. It fails almost as miserably as most primitive human communities, most animals and plants. Japan is almost a unique case in the history of the world.

There can be little doubt that the modifications of species have occurred in much the same way. While proof is impossible, we have the impression that the move forward is sudden, and offensive rather than defensive. We feel that it is not merely the extra pressure of adverse environmental influences which stimulates to mutation; on the contrary, as we have seen, this generally fails to take place. The move forward, the offensive which is taken, usually has a character corresponding to existing living enemies or natural adverse conditions, but it has *élan*. Naturalists indeed, are obliged to assume in many instances that modification has overshot the mark, to the point of producing changes actually opposed to survival. The horns of the stag-beetle and the antlers of the stag are often cited as examples of this.

If we accept mutation as the mechanism of organic development in the lower animals, we are almost compelled to regard invention in man as its psychical correlative, in exactly the same way that Dr. Marston's four primary emotions are the psychical correlatives of the four types of response to stimulus by living matter.[1]

[1] Dr. Marston deals with the creative activity of man, and here I cannot follow him. He regards the commonly drawn comparison between the "creation" of a child by a woman, and that of a work of science, invention or art as sound, since each is the manufacture of a new individual from dead matter. But, of course, the production of a child is *reproduction*, not creation, and analogous to the reproduction of technical objects, scientific experiments, and works of art. The new born individual is only unique, and hence entirely new to the world from a statistical point of view as a chance combination of innumerable genes. The truly new individual is a mutation possessing a gene or genes of a new kind.

In view of the apparent certitude of Weismann's theory it is clear that the discovery of the connection between mutation and invention will present very great difficulties. It may turn out that, although the normal *soma* has no power whatever to modify the germ-plasm which it carries, the abnormal or creative *soma* has this power. The new idea, inoculated into the individual germ plasm in the case of lower organisms, is introduced into the race mind via the consciousness in the case of man and higher animals—the race mind again being the correlative of the undying germ plasm. There is, of course, no need for the original idea ever to be conscious to its creator at all. In the case of mutation in the lower animals, there is no consciousness, as far as we know, to be aware of it. But in the case of man, the actual execution of a new idea may be equally unconscious. In the typical "inspiration" state, the consciousness, so far as it is present, is merely a spectator ; the execution of the work is directed immediately by the unconscious. It cannot be too strongly emphasized that the most brilliant and impressive piece of constructive work, no matter upon what scale, and the creation of a single really new thing, no matter how insignificant are phenomena entirely different in quality. The actual creative invention is notoriously, more often than not, the product of a mind almost pitiably devoid of the range and power of consciousness necessary for sound construction.

These remarks may seem very speculative ; they are already verging on notions such as those of Butler, Hering, Jung and others, which are at present regarded by experimental scientific workers as idle if amusing dreams. But experimental research is actually busy along a whole number of different lines of approach, Freud studies the human unconscious, and finds the *libido*, closely allied to the sex-drive ; Jung finds the race mind. We have seen that mutations of the genes and human invention are closely analogous, and that the latter is generated in the unconscious. Everyone knows Butler's long sight into the future of biological speculation quoted above, and the later development of his line of thought by Hering and Semon. The investigation of the psychology of highly originative human types shows them to be generally abnormal and not far removed from psychopaths—again indicating a peculiar organization of the unconscious. These various facts point to a definite connection between the germ plasm and its reproductive drive—if the *soma* as a rule seems to have no power to modify the germ plasm, the latter through the hormones most certainly acts upon the *soma*—the unconscious, with its libido characteristics ; and the power of origination, which seems to be connected with an abnormal unconscious.

Before leaving the subject, one point of experimental importance may be emphasized. Much experiment is in progress with a view to testing the inheritance of acquired characteristics from other points of view than the mere cutting-off of the tails of mice.

It is hoped that the inheritance of acquired psychical characteristics, or at least aptitudes, may be proved or disproved and that it may even be possible to produce mutations by continually exposing animals to a situation exciting the desire for a certain modification. But if we are right, these experiments have little prospect of success. A negative result would prove nothing. A positive result is extremely unlikely.

For if we place a number of animals in such a position that a certain unfulfilled need, the fulfilment of which requires an adaptation of structure or habit new to the race, is constantly present to them, the chances of this adaptation being made are, as all biology teaches us, extremely small. Most living species, indeed, are exactly in this position. Most races of primitive man are in it— indeed, it is not too much to say that most men and women around us to-day are in the same case. To use a vulgar but expressive phrase, it seems as if they

" haven't the sense to come in out of the rain ". Think
only of the history of the art of warfare up to the
introduction of gun-powder. The invention of the
Welsh long-bow is said by historians to have changed
the face of European history. Examine bows and arrows
of any other kind whatever, and you are astonished
at their feebleness.

It is evident that what is at present beyond our reach
is the production of the forward drive which leads to
modification or invention. The need alone will not
stimulate it. The same fact is impressed upon us by
the observation of our fellow beings.

Meanwhile, it is the task of psychology to elucidate
thoroughly the mental processes, and all their
concomitants, which are peculiar to invention in its
widest sense. The correlative of M. Montmasson's
study is the investigation from a practical and experimental point of view of men of original genius. So far,
the results have been rather disappointing. It is difficult
to see what characteristics of men of genius have been
revealed by the studies of Freudian and other
psychologists, which are not shared by other and quite
unproductive personalities. Whatever be the truth or
otherwise of Freud's study of Leonardo da Vinci, for
instance, it does not tell us, or even pretend to tell us,
in what way this prince of original minds differed from
common men.

We may advert to one theory which, though older
than Freud, is given a definite experimental basis by
his work. This theory states that original genius depends
not so much upon the abnormal powers of forming
combinations in the unconscious. We all possess this
power ; some of the advocates of this theory regard the
unconscious as limitless in extent and in some mystical
way in contact with a Universal Mind. The consciousness
of the genius, however, is freely open to the promptings
and suggestions of the Unconscious, while the normal
person, as Freud has shown, erects an almost impenetrable

barrier, which represses all material which does not conform to a certain specification. Freudians have studied almost exclusively the moral specification, but there is no reason to assume that the mechanism of repression is exclusively moral in nature. The words " right " and " wrong " are used freely in art, science, technology, and every other branch of human conduct, as in morals. We are taught the " right " way to do a thing ; and the man who has learned that the right way to make a steam engine is Newcomen's way, is likely to have a mind closed to a suggestion from his unconscious that the condensing spray need not be in the cylinder of the engine, but might be in a separate compartment. Watt's mind was not thus closed. Many minds must have considered, even consciously, Einstein's fundamental notions, and have rejected them. His genius lay in accepting them and being willing to devote time and energy to testing them.

There is probably a certain amount of truth in this theory. But its applicability is obviously limited. Some original ideas are repulsive to normal minds in their strangeness, but others, equally valuable, are sure of an instantaneous welcome. In the narrow field of technical invention, in which the law has found itself obliged, much to its august discomfort, to decide upon the presence or absence of original inventive power, we are accustomed to the case of a problem which has baffled engineers for years, and is finally solved by a simple means which seems entirely natural and obvious the moment it is stated. What is the peculiarity of the mind which finds such a solution to an old problem ? Such solutions are, of course, found by accident, constantly. But when they are found first in the form of an idea that occurs to a certain mind, that mind is nearly always one characterized by originality, one which also produces inventions not of the simple and obvious kind. It is incredible that, in such cases, the simple solution had existed as an unconscious idea in the minds of all those who had been confronted with the problem, but had been rejected. The law, accordingly, assumes the existence of inventive ingenuity to be proved if the fact that others have tried and failed is proved, no matter how simple the solution.

Apart from this single theory, which appears to be too simple, there exists nothing but a great deal of psychological morphology concerning persons of original genius. While Mr. Montmasson deals with the normal case of the genius with a passion of interest for his life's work, coupled, sometimes but not always, with a passion for distinction, recognition, and worldly reward, we are also confronted with a number of cases where first-rate originality has been displayed almost casually, as a kind of sideline, playfully in a dilettante manner. We have such cases as Pepys in literature, Priestly and Franklin in science.

Then we have the *homò unius libri*, the person who rises to the height of originality once only in an otherwise undistinguished life-time.

Let us return to the normal type of man or woman of genius. Undoubtedly one almost universal characteristic is that of a passionate interest in a certain field or work. The genius is nearly always in love with his work, or at any rate obsessed by it. The analogy with sexual passion is a close one ; for there, too, the obsession with one object is coloured with joy for one person, with bitterness for another. The genius is rarely, however, of the one-idea'd type, and there are thousands of unoriginal minds whose whole interest in life is narrowed to one single field, for one genius of that kind. Normally, the genius is a man of great energy and many potentialities, which are only neglected regretfully in the service of the grand passion.

The origin of this grand passion is surely a matter susceptible of psychological investigation. We not uncommonly meet with people whose power and energy impress us to the point of believing that nothing but the absence of a dominant interest in any single branch of activity is wanting to make them take rank with genius. Although we meet also with men who have all the classic characteristics of original genius except the genius, but including the passion, it would still be worth while to know whether such passion is inborn or implanted, and if so, how. We might even hope to implant it of set purpose. This would almost certainly have to be done before the fifth to seventh years of life. In all probability it should be done, if at all, by selecting some physically attractive individual of real or pretended great fame, and having him do something impressive and spectacular in his own line of work, in personal contact with the child.

Another matter for investigation is the attitude of the genius towards the object of his passion. The passion of the non-genius is characterized by an immense satisfaction in the glories and powers of his subject. He is rather like the lover who can see no defects whatever in his mistress. It is thus that the nineteenth century teacher of physics and other sciences, full of passion for his subject, left his young charges in ignorance of all those skeletons in the cupboard, the rattle of whose bones was inspiration to the men of genius who have revolutionized our science. The genius, on the other hand, is either benevolently or malevolently critical. If benevolent, he desires to carry on where others have left off ; he sees the ragged end, the vacant plot upon which to build. If malevolent he doubts, doubts the work of past investigators and the teaching of accepted doctrinaires. He loves his subject, but is always jealous of those in the past who have been wedded to it.

We see almost analogous attitudes in the love of man for woman ; whole-hearted, uncritical admiration ; an almost pædagogic desire to help, improve, train, develop ; or finally, a rather bitter critical attitude desiring to unmake, if possible, and remake. It is not in the least improbable that Freudian psychology could already tell us a great deal which would explain these various attitudes in both cases.

The fact that a person may have all the characteristics of original genius excepting the power of producing new ideas applies, apparently, even to the subjective sensations of the subject. This is not so self-evident in science and technology, since a false sensation of inspiration can only arise when a false idea is produced, and such ideas are usually quickly disproved. But this is not always the case, and we have a few contemporary cases of men of high attainments who have produced worthless, although apparently recondite ideas, with all the appearance of triumphant action. But in art, literature, sociology, and so on, such cases are numerous indeed. Writers produce prose and poetry of the most commonplace description with a finer frenzy, probably, than Shakespeare or Goethe : indeed, the latter himself remarked upon this fact.

The conclusion seems inescapable that, apart from all other concomitants, creation requires a specific creative faculty. It remains for psychologists to track this to its lair in the unconscious, and to find out, if possible, whether it occurs at all times and places, in all human beings remaining undeveloped, atrophied or inactive in all human beings, most of the time, and in most all the time.

For all the complexity of the subject, the definition of the quest is simple. A human being feels a need—to express himself to others, to understand phenomena, to clothe, feed, transport himself, fight others, communicate at a distance with his kind, and what not. To satisfy this need he uses successfully means other than those which he has been taught : different words, different colours, forms and sounds, different theories and explanations, different tools, devices, materials, stratagems, and so forth. Different *and* successful. This person's mind is a rare and special case, and it is a very important matter for psychology to investigate this case.

We now come to another set of psychological problems, of equal moment, upon which M. Montmasson does not touch. These are problems of mass-psychology. When invention is active, there is not only a problem presented by the minds which originate, but also by those, the vast majority, which incorporate the new ideas, more or less quickly, into their own stock.

At first sight conservatism requires no explanation. For all our rapid progress in the past few centuries, we are fully familiar with it. We find, indeed, that every community known to us shows a greater or less proportion of persons who actively or passively resist every change in their ideas, methods, or habits. We can find individual farmers, manufacturers, shopkeepers, and so on, alive to-day and interviewable by anyone, who exemplify in their own persons the general biological rule that destruction is preferred to modification. In parts of the world, such as America, where white civilization is spreading rapidly, some aboriginal or primitive races are fading away sullenly, ceasing to multiply, losing their vitality, while others are adapting themselves quite joyfully to the changed conditions. Surely it is conservatism, which in these cases amounts to suicide, that requires psychological investigation.

But conservatism in these cases resists the plain, demonstrable logic of coming in out of the wet. We see, at any rate, how hopeless must be the case of the would-be innovator in normal, stable communities. We do not need to assume that the faculty of creation is missing in these. The sheer force of conservatism would be ample to crush it. In communities in a state of living and developing culture, on the other hand, the force of conservatism is but a brake on the wheel, which rolls on. It should be noted, also, that this development is not, as a whole, in the nature of adaptation to changed and menacing conditions; it is not defence, but offence. On the other hand, the majority of individuals are placed in the position of having to adapt themselves or go under. Conservatism in the vast majority results in a wastage, but also, to some extent, is beneficial by preventing changes being made too rapidly or prematurely.

The really intriguing thing is the psychology of the ruling and determining elements. The beginning of a culture is probably, in all cases, signalized by the rise of a new religious belief. Here psychological study has been, and will continue to be, busy. The conservative, traditional character of the primitive community is shaken, and the ruler or rulers are bound to incorporate the new religious movement, and hence to abandon tradition. Very soon, development is in full march. From the first, there is a demand for invention and elaboration. A theology and policy are developed, there is a call for art. Most strangely, originality is least in demand in connection with the useful arts. When we consider the rapid development of the few centuries preceding Roger Bacon the opposition which he met with is truly astonishing.

The fundamental characteristic seems to be that most of the powerful members of the community are in need of new ideas, which they can utilize to enhance their own power or diminish that of their rivals. This state of affairs would appear to be almost essential to the progress of human invention. Nothing could be more certain than that the inventor entirely lacks the power of " putting it over ". This process is always accomplished by " appetitive " types (Marston). I might add at this point that, while I have ventured to differ from Dr. Marston on one point, his main conclusions, also in regard to originative workers, appear to me entirely sound. The original genius is undoubtedly what he calls a " love type ", and his classification of human types is altogether a most important advance in psychology.

According to Dr. Marston, the primary emotion " dominance " is characteristic of the appetitive type. It represents the response of living matter to a stimulus felt as hostile. Such a stimulus may be met either by " dominance " or " compliance ", by fighting or by running away. It is clear from our analysis that inventive change needs dominance to enable it to survive.

Biologically, the various emotional responses to stimulus may be finally determined by hormonic or other chemical balances. Such is the assumption of a whole school of human physiological psychology. It may be, therefore, that the power and impulse to produce new and useful modifications is always and everywhere present in living organisms, and that the decisive factor which leads to advance or modification is a chemical change corresponding to changing the balance of response to stimulus in favour of dominance. The rise and development of a civilization might thus finally depend upon a change in the endocrine balance of a section of mankind, and since this rise appears to be a matter rather of a certain geographical area than of the races of man living therein, perhaps the change might simply be due to a change in climatic influences, or even a subtle change in diet. The sudden disappearance of the scent of the musk-plant all over the world simultaneously indicates the kind of possibility which cannot be left out of account.

We may now leave the reader to M. Montmasson's remarkable study, hoping that what has been here said may recur to him from time to time and stimulate thought in the direction of further research.

H. STAFFORD HATFIELD.

INVENTION AND THE
UNCONSCIOUS

INTRODUCTION

A FACT has struck me : the first idea of a large number
of inventions was not the logical outcome of long
trains of reasoning ; it was revealed suddenly to the mind
of the seeker, after a long *unconscious* incubation.

I should like first of all to define the extent of this
unconscious elaboration by drawing a clear distinction
between what is conscious and what is not. I shall then
endeavour to explain, by known laws of psychology
and by a theory of consciousness which I believe to be
somewhat novel, this silent action of the unconscious
in the genesis of invention.

What is the *Unconscious* ? What is *Invention* in
general ? What is *scientific invention* in particular ?
These words must be defined with great precision if it is
desired to gain a clear idea of the problem which will
be enunciated in the following pages : *What is the rôle
of the Unconscious in Scientific Invention ?*

I. THE UNCONSCIOUS

The term *unconscious* is negative ; it is like cold as
related to heat, night as related to day. But we understand heat better than cold, day better than night.

Therefore, in order to get a clear grasp of the meaning of the word *unconscious*, let us study first of all the meaning of the term *consciousness*.

(a) The Study of the Unconscious should be preceded by an analysis and a definition of the Consciousness

Some psychologists maintain that nothing is more indefinable than consciousness. Is it not " inherent in the phenomena which accompany it " ?[1] If I think, if I wish, if I suffer, am I not also, at the same moment, conscious of my thought, of my desire, of my suffering ? Now to define consciousness would be to distinguish it from the phenomenon to which it is bound ; that would be, so Leibniz thought, not only to feel and to be conscious of feeling, but also to be conscious of being conscious.[2] Is not that a tautology ? In no way. The facts alleged simply prove that the consciousness, which is coextensive with our several mental states, is not a special faculty, as Reid, Jouffroy, Garnier, Royer-Collard imagined it to be ; they do not show that a definition of consciousness is impossible ; but a definition of this kind should precisely express those characters of generality and inwardness which conscious knowledge presents. I feel myself existing and I am conscious of my *being* ; I perceive the *pleasure* or *pain* in me ; I experience *feelings, sensations, volitions* ; I have ideas of *unity, simplicity,* and *identity*, for I am a unique subject, mysteriously identical under the diverse vicissitudes of my existence ; I find in the continuity of my activity the idea of *duration,* in the succession of phenomena the relations of anterior and posterior which constitute the concept of *time* ; if I compare my states of consciousness, I have the idea of *difference* ; if I count them, I have the idea of *number* ; if I consider myself as the permanent subject of phenomena, the changing picture of which I see pass

---

[1] P.-F. Thomas, *Cours de philosophie*, Paris, 1921, p. 21.
[2] Quoted by Fouillée, *L'évolutionisme des idées-forces*, p. 37.

before me, I am conscious of being a *substance*; I feel myself capable of effort, of power, and am thus a *cause*; I act with a definite end in view and thus arrive at the idea of *purpose*; if I act in one sense, I know that I could choose to act in the opposite sense—that is the idea of *liberty*; finally, I stand proudly upright and feel myself a force which is enlightened and master of its acts. I have the idea of my body and the continual and vague sensation of its action upon me (cenæsthesia), I have the idea of my character, that is, my usual manner of feeling, thinking and wishing: I have the idea of *personality* or the idea of my *ego*.[1]

In short, this analysis reveals to me consciousness, or the internal perception of a series of coexistent or successive states. What I know thus are my pleasures, my thoughts, my desires: consciousness is thus *personal* consciousness. The ideas concerning my internal states are given me without any intermediary: consciousness is thus *direct* knowledge. In this sanctuary of my mind, shut off from any indiscreet inspection by a stranger consciousness, I am alone in seeing myself in this or that light: for consciousness is *impenetrable*.

The combination of these various characteristics enables us to give the following definition of consciousness, a definition the exactness and generality of which will suffice to help to a subsequent delimitation of the field of the unconscious :—

Consciousness is the immediate, spontaneous, or reflective knowledge of the internal states and phenomena of the mind by the mind itself and by the mind alone.

(b) Consciousness has limits

This definition allows us to trace the frontiers of consciousness. Must we suppose, with Hamilton, that consciousness, being coextensive with our faculties, is limited by these faculties themselves ? That would be to affirm that we are conscious of our body, of the external

[1] Sortais, *Manuel de philosophie*, Paris, 1907, pp. 80-2.

world, of God, of the past and future, since we know our body, the world, God, the past, and, to some extent, the future. Deplorable confusion! My consciousness is personal; I cannot escape from its proper domain. Hence, if I know the object A, I am not conscious of A, which is external to me, I am simply conscious that, in fact, I know A; I am conscious, not of A, but of my knowledge of A. In that respect my consciousness does not leave its territory, which is entirely interior. That being so, I have no consciousness of my own body, contrary to the opinion of Maine de Biran, but I am conscious of internal muscular and vital sensations which serve in my case as intermediaries between the conscious interior and the external body. Nor am I any more conscious of the physiological transformations of which my body is the theatre, but I receive from them the repercussion of sensations which are truly conscious. Am I better informed by consciousness concerning the external world? Not in the least: for I only know of its existence and of its qualities through the sensations which it causes in me. The same exclusion holds good for the past, the future, the absolute, the infinite, and God himself: I am only conscious of the idea of God, of the idea of the absolute, of the idea of infinity, of the idea of the future, and the idea of the past.

(c) Consciousness is related to sensibility

Sensation is thus the necessary intermediary between the consciousness and the external world. But sensation arises partly from sensibility and partly from intelligence, since it is at once affective and representative. We thus have consciousness, thanks to sensation, linked with sensibility.

But what is sensibility? " The faculty of being affected painfully or agreeably by all interior and exterior causes." [1] But pleasure and pain are related to consciousness. We do not need here to investigate whether

---

[1] Dumont, *Théorie scientifique de la sensibilité*, Paris, 1875, p. 25.

knowledge precedes the feeling or whether the feeling precedes consciousness (of it). Let us simply take note that, for a large number of philosophers, the affective phenomenon is accompanied by the intellectual phenomenon of consciousness.

For Descartes, in fact, pleasure and pain are proportional to the knowledge of our perfections or our imperfections; for Spinoza, sadness is the feeling of our impotence (the word feeling here designating a confused knowledge); this is also the opinion of Leibniz, for whom " pleasure and pain arise from confused representations which make known to us the increase or decrease in our vitality ". Kant defines pleasure as " the consciousness of vital effort " ; for Wolf, " pleasure depends upon the confused knowledge of some perfection " ; for Vivès, " pleasure is a relation of agreement between the faculties and their object." According to Herbart, " pleasure is the tension of a representation more favoured than opposed " ; Grote defines feeling as " the conscious product of an unconscious estimation of certain relations ". Hegel in the same sense, " feeling is a confused knowledge." For Dumont, " pleasure is the knowledge of a composition of forces." Finally Fouillée, who collects all these statements, condenses his own thought in these terms : " to enjoy or to suffer is to feel oneself living more or less ; perception precedes, accompanies, or follows feeling ; in all enjoyment there is a ray of intellectual discernment." [1]

(d) Consciousness and Sensibility as related to force

One could not better characterize the close bond which unites consciousness to sensibility.

But Dumont, who is followed by Fouillée, goes further. For them, consciousness is connected with force.

According to Dumont, indeed, " consciousness is force taken subjectively, the intimate state of force ; but each force is only conscious on its own account ;

[1] Fouillée, *Psychologie des idées-forces*, Paris, 1893, vol. i, p. 98.

Consciousness changes at every modification of force. Under these conditions pleasure is the consciousness of a composition of forces, pain, the consciousness of a diminution of force." [1]

Hartmann thinks that " force does not become conscious excepting in the case when it meets another force and is modified by it ".[2] Dumont goes further : " every force is conscious alike of its permanent states and of its changes of state. At every change of state the same consciousness is agreeably or disagreeably affected, according as the change is to greater or to less." [3]

Fouillée is of the same opinion : " ideas may be idea-forces ; ideas are the forms not only of thought but of wishes ; they are acts conscious of their exertion, of their direction, of their quality, and of their intensity.

But this force is not simply latent energy. Dumont and Fouillée picture it to themselves under the form of movement : " ideas are motors," says Fouillée, " sensation, pleasure and pain correspond to an increase, a decrease, or a displacement of the forces of the organism ; sensation is not a force added to movement : it is an aspect of movement." Fouillée adds to this statement of Dumont another which it is interesting to record : " The transformation of potential force into living force and movement causes pleasure : all normal and proportioned action causes enjoyment ; pleasure and pain are related to life : to enjoy or to suffer is to feel oneself living more or less."

Thus consciousness, already connected with sensibility is thus again connected with force. But, taking a thought of Leibniz's, Dumont deduces the following consequence from it : " As in the totality of the Universe the amount of force remains constant, so too is the amount of pleasure or pain constant." We may also draw this conclusion from it : pleasure or pain, the form of sensibility or of

---

[1] Dumont, op. cit., p. 64.
[2] Quoted by Dumont, ibid.
[3] Ibid.

consciousness may vary; but the force represented by this consciousness will remain identical. This constant dynamic, the true living force of sensibility, will be utilized in the second part of this study.

(e) Consciousness reinforced by attention

Whether it is connected with sensibility, or reduced to a form of mental energy, consciousness appears to us with a certain tonality, a certain degree of concentration, that is, *attention*.

If I analyse this mental operation I see first of all the act by which it stops at one object to the exclusion of others; for there is produced in me a momentary arrest of sensations and ideas; there then follows an actual tension towards one or several definite ideas. It is not absolutely " one-ideadness " as Ribot affirms; but it is a considerable contraction of the field of my consciousness: it is an effect analogous to the action of a convergent lens. The points of which I was previously only vaguely conscious because they seemed to be a discontinuous series, have approached one another to such an extent that they give the impression of a continuous straight line, but one shorter than before. The two adjoining figures illustrate the difference between dispersed and attentive consciousness.

```
1.  Dispersed consciousness
    ▬ ▬ ▬ ▬ ▬ ▬ ▬

2.  Attention (1st degree)
    ............................

    Attention (2nd degree)
    ─────────────
```

Psychologists have given these different degrees of attention separate names: *distraction, contemplation, application, meditation, contention*. In place of a series of luminous points, I gradually obtain a luminous train similar to the golden dust left behind upon their paths by shooting stars. In every case, these fractions of consciousness appear to be drawn toward one another, joined by cohesion or rather by affinity, adhering together in such manner as to give the impression of a single idea. What is the origin of this cement, what is the cause of this concentratioh ?

Fouillée and Ribot suppose that it is interest. They are right ; affective states explain all degrees of attention. Teachers, to be convinced of this, have only to remember that the best way to teach is to excite the interest of their pupils in order to hold their attention. On the other hand, the will also plays an important part in this genesis of the attention. " Attention," says Fouillée, " is the intellectual reaction under the influence of a desire or a volition." [1] This double source, sensibility and will, allows us to explain both spontaneous and voluntary attention.

On the strength of these observations, Fouillée is able to say " attention is consciousness itself, the consciousness of oneself seizing itself in its reaction to external impressions : in attention, a fact has, on account of it, more concomitants able to connect it for an instant with the general content of consciousness . . . It weakens the force of representation from which it turns away, and adds force to the ideas upon which it concentrates : *it prolongs the state of consciousness to which it applies itself* ".[2]

(*f*) *As a result of attention, we pass from consciousness to the unconscious*

Thus consciousness, already defined by the ideas of *personal knowledge, sensibility*, and *force*, also implies the concept of *attention*. What is the exact part played by this idea ? Comparisons will assist us to characterize

---

[1] Fouillée, op. cit., vol. i, p. 309.
[2] Op. cit., vol. i, p. 221.

it. We have a clear idea of the temperature, of the degree of heat of a body—of electrical potential, the level of the electric fluid in a conductor—of an algebraic coefficient, the multiplier of any quantity. We then say : Attention is like the *temperature* of consciousness, the potential of consciousness, the coefficient of consciousness.

Consciousness, on account of the part played by attention, will thus pass through all degrees, and hence through zero. At the limit of its decrease, the consciousness will be zero. What does that mean ? It will be a psychical phenomenon, a consciousness, since, right through the series, we have to do with consciousness. But the degree of this consciousness is zero, and hence this term of consciousness refers to a psychical fact to which I pay no attention at all, a real activity but one totally ignored by the *ego*, a real mental state, but one the transformations of which take place entirely without my knowledge. In short, this consciousness measured by zero attention becomes the unconscious. The theory of attention considered in consciousness allows us to pass from consciousness to the unconscious.

M. J. Jastrow explains in the same way as we do the decrease of consciousness by the progressive disappearance of attention. "A message is brought to the mind by the senses. Three acts are to be distinguished in this process : *reception, interpretation*, and *expression*. Inattention to one of these three acts diminishes consciousness in two ways : by weakening the *sensation* and by ignorance of the *origin* of an impression which it experiences. A mother, for example, asks her daughter to bring her a certain book. The child is absentminded, fails to answer, and does not move. A moment afterwards, it brings the book and says, "Mother, I saw your book *by chance* and thought that you perhaps would like to have it." The girl executes an order received without having been conscious of its reception.[1]

---

[1] J. Jastrow, *La subconscience*, translated by Philippi, Paris, 1908, pp. 91-3.

(g) *The Unconscious Exists*

The unconscious exists as the residue of a consciousness which has reached its minimum of attention. The fact is certain. I can prove it in the memory : a multitude of my ideas have been preserved in it without my knowledge. It appears in perception : if it be too weak, too strong, or too often repeated, an impression remains imperceptible. I find it in certain cases of the *association of ideas* : the sight of the *Gioconda* in the Louvre at once causes me to think of one of my dead comrades. At first I am ignorant of the reason. Upon reflexion, the cause is revealed : this school-friend had developed at that time the portrait of the illustrious Florentine. My purely intellectual operations : judgments, generalizations, reasonings even, are often unconscious in origin : my dislike of certain people, my prejudices, my tastes, my instinctive preferences cannot be logically explained by the immediate antecedents of my thought. Finally, my instinctive movements, my habits, my repeated volitions, a great deal of my activity and my sensibility are ruled by the unconscious.

(h) *Theories of the Nature of the Unconscious*

The unconscious exists. But what is the nature of it ? The opinions on this question can be divided into three groups : (1) Theories relating to the *impersonal* or *metaphysical* unconscious ; (2) Hypotheses of the *distant* or *palingenetic* unconscious ; (3) The various conceptions of the *psychological, personal* unconscious.

(1) Aristotle, with his doctrine of the νους ποιητικὸς which he also calls νους χωριστὸς, appears to admit a certain unconscious activity, distinctive of the organism ; the active intellect, impassive, immaterial, is immortal with an immortality which is mingled with that of the divine intelligence.[1]

Plotinus is already more precise : " We are always

---

[1] Aristotle; *De anima*, bk. iii, ch. v.

thinking," he says, "but we do not always think one thought : the most noble effort of the mind is to lose itself in unity with the principle of intelligence. The highest knowledge is unconscious."

For Fichte, the Divine Being is unconscious knowledge—it tends to become absolute consciousness by dividing itself into a multitude of individual consciousnesses.[1]

Schelling shows us the creation of the world by the unconscious. "Nothing prevents me from going back to a moment when this ego, which is now fully conscious of itself, was not yet fully conscious of its being. For the absolute ego, in its phase of unconsciousness, produced external things . . . The unconscious thinks in us and acts in Nature. This force realizes a world which it does not know."

This realization is viewed by Hegel in another manner. He distinguishes three stages in the passage from the unconscious to the conscious ; the first period is that of absolute unconsciousness ; here the idea in itself is considered. In the second, we pass from the idea to consciousness ; in the third, finally, we reach absolute consciousness ; the idea is grasped again in unity. The divine Spirit works in the artist ; consciousness is a progress.

Schopenhauer, as opposed to Hegel, regards consciousness as an evil. The unconscious principle of things is a will. The idea cannot exist before the object : the thing in itself comes first ; it is a force, the will.

The universal will is unconscious ; for consciousness is a phenomenon, and therefore has an accidental character. The unconscious will has arrived at consciousness, thanks to an organ which is the brain in the higher animals. Through it the world becomes a representation.[2]

Hartmann, finally, who inherits Schopenhauer's

---

[1] Quoted by Hartmann, *Philosophy of the Unconscious*, vol. i, p. 25.

[2] Schopenhauer, *Die Welt als Wille und Vorstellung, passim.*

thought, transforms it in order to make it, as he thinks, a definite philosophy of consciousness. For him, the unconscious thought is eternal; he, also, thinks that consciousness appeared with the brain. He reasons as follows. The intelligence which rules everything is substantially identical with the world, but the manifestations of this spiritual force are diverse : vivifying and curative action in a sick body ; reflex movements ; the unconscious execution of movements which accompany voluntary action ; formation of feelings, evolution of character, etc. Now conscious thought cannot explain the recall of memories, nor the latent reasoning which leads to the recognition of an object, nor the operations of abstraction and generalization, nor all the *a priori* categories of thought which pre-exist in consciousness, nor, finally, æsthetic judgments which are formed without our knowing how. Hence it is necessary to admit as anterior to all knowledge, a universal unconscious, the silent action of which takes account of all the preceding facts. Hence, in Hartmann also we find the passage from the impersonal unconscious to individual consciousness.

(2) In Plato we find the germs of the distant or palingenetic unconscious. For him, indeed, the perceptions of the senses are the recollections of ideas known to souls before their union with bodies. Now these particular souls arise by emanation from the cosmic soul or God. The theory of reminiscence implies a certain unconscious participation by the soul in Divine truth. The actual conscious soul is, as it were, a degradation of the Divine principle from which, unknowingly, it derives its origin. It is this primitive existence, this distant unconsciousness, which explains the doctrine of reminiscence.[1]

Dr. Geley, for another reason, supports the theory of palingenesis. His reasoning is as follows. The facts

[1] Cf. Piat, *Platon*, ch. v, pp. 167, 173, 174. M. Huit has, however, cast doubt upon the accuracy of this interpretation in the *Bulletin Critique*, April, 1907, pp. 178–9.

produced by unconscious psychical activity are innumerable and often marvellous: cryptamnesia, mental suggestion, telepathy, etc. Now these facts and, in general the whole unconscious memory, appear to be independent of cerebral contingencies : they pass beyond the bounds of actual consciousness. Hence, the experiences of the present life do not account for a part of the subconscious : the rest must be explained by past lives.

Thus, actual consciousness, by virtue of the whole subconscious memory, would come from the distant unconscious. Hindu philosophers, with their doctrine of metempsychosis, can readily subscribe to this doctrine, which the author is careful to call a metaphysical hypothesis.

(3) The psychological unconscious appears to have been supported by St. Augustine in the fourth century. In his *Confessions* he expresses himself thus : " Our soul cannot embrace its whole extension, nor its whole essence." [1] Is this not a recognition of the fact that the soul is incompletely conscious, that its faculties surpass the limits of consciousness ? But it also affirms that this domain of the unexplored soul is not foreign to it. There is an unconscious, but a personal unconscious.

This theory is carried further by Leibniz ; for him, " thought is the representation of the multiple in the simple." But the representation is a correspondence of analogous states. Thus thought is the representation of these analogous states, that is to say, the representation of the multiple in the simple. This representation is the apanage of all beings ; unconscious perceptions only differ in degree from clear apperceptions : thus thought is the universal act of things. There are beings who have conscious perceptions and those that have unconscious perceptions ; man has both. Unconscious are the virtualities or innate principles of reason ; these are the intellectual instincts. Unconscious are the unnoticed

[1] *Confessions*, vol. x, ch. 8.

perceptions of our vital activity. Unconscious, a thousand perceptions of which the result alone is perceived. Unconscious are the ideas which are preserved in memory and afterwards reappear. Unconscious are the latent influences which act on the will. Now there is identity between activity and perception. By virtue of the law of continuity, one must admit more or less conscious perceptions between consciousness and the unconscious. The absolute unconscious is the limit.

This doctrine was taken up and partly modified by Hamilton. This philosopher reserves the term *consciousness* for thought endowed with a certain intensity. However, if this intensity is below a certain minimum, unconscious states and acts are possible. They are, in fact, numerous and various : items of knowledge of which we do not actually think ; systems of knowledge which are only revealed to consciousness in certain moments of extraordinary exaltation, such as the recollections of certain invalids ; active or passive states of the mind— unconscious in themselves—but manifesting their activity by conscious effects, like small unconscious perceptions of which the sum-total of perception is constant, or the apparent gaps in the chain of our association of ideas, linked by unconscious intermediate steps. Here is the general theory of this author : suppose that the ideas *A* and *C* cannot suggest one another, but that both are associated with the idea *B*. It may happen that we are conscious of *A* and immediately afterwards of *C*. How are we to explain these anomalies ? By the principle of latent modifications. I thought of *A* consciously, and *B* suggested *C* to me. If *B*, which served as the track uniting the two, remained unconscious, it is because this idea was below the minimum perceptible.[1]

Stuart Mill does not admit this ingenious explanation. ' What is unconscious,' he thinks, ' is not the idea, but the simple power of thinking afresh. Everyone knows

[1] Hamilton, *Lectures*, vol. i, pp. 339, 352, 353.

that we have faculties of which we are not conscious; but these are only aptitudes for receiving impressions.' Mill replaces the intermediary unconscious by nervous modifications. He does not admit the existence of unconscious perceptions.

The unconscious life, which is very important in the eyes of Hamilton, becomes preponderant for Maudsley. According to him, consciousness is only an epiphenomenon, or witness. The essential activity is unconscious activity. Consciousness, in this view, is injurious to the mind's activity.

But, in a train of reasoning, what are the unconscious, and what are the conscious elements? Wundt teaches us that if the reasoning is conscious, the premises and the conclusion are conscious. But in perception, the premises are unconscious states; hence the antecedents of the train of reasoning escape consciousness; the conclusion alone is conscious. The author does not suppose that totally unconscious reasoning exists, as others have thought.

This delimitation of the field of the unconscious is conceived by Herbart in another manner. He thinks that all psychical phenomena are intellectual in nature. Under these conditions, the actual representation are conscious : only the tendencies to representations are unconscious. There is never a rigorous solution of continuity beween the consciousness and the unconscious; psychical life is, in fact, a perpetual oscillation of perceptions which descend below the threshold of consciousness and of perceptions which rise above it. This incessant coming and going arises from the antagonism of representations; some drive out others; those that are driven out tend to return to their places. Such resemblance as exists between them constitutes the general idea, the permanent residue, which is apparently unconscious, but formed little by little from conscious elements. Thus, on account of this uninterrupted flux and reflux, there is continuity between thoughts in action, and potential

INTRODUCTION

ᵢthoughts : between the domains of the conscious and the unconscious there is only a difference of degree.[1]

This explanation, which is certainly very ingenious, inspired the beautiful essay of Colsenet on the unconscious life of the spirit. According to him, the work of the unconscious in creating associations, and determining groupings, takes place according to the laws of conscious intelligence, but it is more active and certain, since it is performed without distraction. Hence the unconscious is not the Divine Spirit acting within us, but simply the latent working of the human mind. In memory, in the emotions, we have as it were, an idea begun, an unconscious idea.[2]

Desdouits finds this estimate of the domain of the unconscious much too large. In his opinion it is the forms, and not the acts, of the reason which subsist in the unconscious state : unconscious ideas do not exist, nor do unconscious reasonings or even judgments. The unconscious factors are either the effects of habit, or factors of a physiological order, or the laws of the intelligence. Thus everything in perception is to be referred to consciousness ; the memory itself, in which so large a part has been ascribed to the unconscious, is to be restored to consciousness, since, as Royer Collard says, " we do not remember things : we only remember ourselves," that is to say, our perceptions and conscious emotions. Desdouits does not admit the unconscious in the logical intermediaries which, according to this philosopher, prepare the truths of intuition. The mind thinks by analogy or habit, but every intellectual act is accompanied by consciousness, for every judgment is an affirmation, and presupposes the consciousness of certainty or doubt. Desdouits limits the unconscious to psychical states, tendencies created by habit, and ideas in a provisional state.[3]

[1] Herbart, *Psychologie der Wissenschaft*, introduction.
[2] Colsenet, *La vie inconsciente de l'esprit*, Paris, 1880, pp. 28–111.
[3] Desdouits, *Philosophie de l'inconscient*, Paris, 1892, pp. 108–9.

Dumont holds an equally limited view of the unconscious.[1]

Fouillée sees in the unconscious "only a paralysed consciousness, a consciousness too weak to see what is passing within itself, or an association of weak states of consciousness with strong ones ; or further, only diminutions or displacements of consciousness ".[2]

Dwelshauvers, however, realizes that the facts of the unconscious are too numerous to be treated as exceptions confirming the general law of consciousness. In his large work on the unconscious,[3] he summarizes all the opinions put forward on this subject by his predecessors, and completes the classification of forms of the unconscious. He agrees with Fouillée in rejecting the metaphysical unconscious. He distinguishes a rational unconscious, which orders the impressions of the mind in a logical manner : a psycho-physiological unconscious, comprising the unconscious part of the perceptions : an automatic unconscious, corresponding to the psychological automatism of Janet, and the subconscious of other psychologists. By the term co-conscious the author denotes psychical acts, ideas, and affective states which detach themselves from the ego to form a second personality ; this is the secondary ego of Pierre Morton, the sublimal self or duplicate personality of other authors. He also speaks of the latent active unconscious, comprising ideas, recollections, impulses, which have been repressed and return suddenly to consciousness (Freud's theory of repressions). These are the images which set the inventive imagination and artistic creation to work ; telepathy and clairvoyance are regarded as connected with this unconscious.

Further, we have the memory unconscious, appearing in tendencies and associations of ideas : every present idea is spread out upon this unconscious foundation.

---

[1] Op. cit., pp. 108–9.
[2] Fouillée, op. cit., vol. i, p. 342.
[3] Dwelshauvers, L'inconscient, Paris, 1916.

Then the affective, irrational, or passional unconscious, which prepares our affective states, renders them durable, and fixes them as feelings or passions. Then the hereditary unconscious, consisting in natural proclivities, leading to natural vocations, and producing the inventors, designers, musicians. Finally we have the remarkable fact of the unconscious in consciousness itself : far from being an epiphenomenon, the consciousness is a synthesis issuing from unconscious activity, and rising by way of evolution to full knowledge of itself. Thus its origin is unconscious, and, at various stages of its activity, it retains its unconscious part.

In the following we shall confine ourselves to the personal psychological unconscious, and retain all those forms classified by Dwelshauvers which represent psychical activity not observed by consciousness. We regard them all as derived from conscious activity by progressive diminution of the attention. Hence if, as we have seen, conscious activity is in relation with sensibility and force, unconscious activity ought also to be a form of sensibility, and an aspect of force, for the internal gaze of the consciousness cannot have the power to modify the nature of psychical states.

II. INVENTION AND DISCOVERY

According to the definition given in the Dictionary of the French Academy, "invention is the faculty of invention, the disposition of the mind towards inventing." To invent is to find something new or ingenious, by the power of one's mind, of one's imagination. One invents an art, a science, a system, a machine, a procedure, a means, an expedient, a fashion, a game. Thus, the arts of writing and printing were invented. Finally, the inventive mind is that which has the talent, the genius, of invention. We speak of "an inventive man, an inventive mind, an inventive imagination". Further, the word invention also designates the thing invented : one speaks of the compass and the barometer as inventions. The thing invented may be an art, a science, a theory, a fashion : it is in every case a combination of elements tending towards a certain end.

Littré, in his dictionary of the French language, adds : " invention combines known conditions in a new manner," giving as an example in this connection the invention of gunpowder.

On the other hand, to discover is to take away what covers a thing, to find out something hitherto unknown, something that had remained hidden, ignored. It is to commence to perceive. Thus we discover a mine, a career, a treasure, an unknown country, a secret issue, the hitherto unknown cause of a disease, a new theory. In this sense, Harvey discovered the circulation of the blood. " Discovery " is either the action of discovering or the thing discovered. Its object will be, for example, a treasure, a secret, a principle, a scientific law. We speak of discoveries in physics, in chemistry, in astronomy, as we speak of the discovery of the New World, and of a voyage of discovery.

These two definitions closely resemble one another. To invent is to find something new, and to imagine something ingenious. On the other hand, to discover is to find what is not known. In both cases we are dealing with a novelty, but invention causes it to exist, discovery makes it known. Invention is thus a creation, discovery a revelation. Invention is a combination of known conditions in a novel manner, it is a production. Psychologically, invention is the work of the creative imagination directed by the reason. Discovery has created nothing, has constructed nothing new : but it sees what is new, a very general principle, a germ that will be fertile. But it does not itself make the germ fertile ; psychologically it is the work of the intuitive reason.

This distinction is brought out in the double definition given by Sommer :—

20 INTRODUCTION

"Discovery adds to our knowledge; it belongs to the domain of science. Invention gives us new help, new resources; it belongs to the domain of art."

In reality, invention, as much as discovery, depends upon science. The instance given by Sommer proves this : "the invention of the barometer is due to Pascal." Everyone knows that the barometer is an application of the physical theory of the variation of atmospheric pressure. It is an invention which owes its existence to science. This observation might be extended to many other inventions. But it is accurate to say that in every invention there is a practical end, attained by various combinations. Invention belongs to the domain of both science and art : it participates in both. As a work of science, it is, as it were, the prolongation of discovery, its extended and developed objectivation. Bacon took this view of it, and in his *De augmentis scientiarum* he writes : "the true and legitimate object of the sciences consists solely in endowing human life with new inventions and new riches." He reproaches antiquity "with having invented nothing to ameliorate and improve the lot of humanity".[1] He would have science active and fertile in inventions. Also, he adds, "the first inventors were looked upon as gods."[2] Finally, he defines invention : *Ars quaedam indicii et directionis quae caeteras artes earumque axiomata atque opera delegat et in conspectum det.*[3] This practical science which discovers and makes known the other sciences by revealing their directing principles, partakes both of discovery—since it makes known new principles—and of invention—since it utilizes them in original constructions.

This is also Bouty's opinion.[4] According to him, the industrialist is on the watch for inventions, the scientist for discoveries . . . When an invention does not come

[1] *Nov. Organ.,* i, 1.
[2] *De interpretatione naturae,* vol. iii.
[3] *De augmentis scientiarum,* vol. v, v. 2.
[4] Bouty, *La vérité scientifique, sa poursuite,* Paris, 1908.

about by chance, it is the setting to work of known principles with a practical end in view : it does not constitute a piece of scientific progress, but it prepares for one. An invention has a character of definite actuality.

Nevertheless, says Bouty, certain inventions are discoveries. We give as examples the principle of the cold well of Watt or the coherer of Branly. In mathematics invention is connected with experiment by bonds of all kinds : it is thus distinguished from demonstration, which is essentially rational.[1] In the physical and biological sciences, even more than in mathematics, experimenting favours invention : Claude Bernard tells us that " the experimenter is an inventor of phenomena and a true foreman of creation ". Finally, in current speech discovery and invention are closely related, since, according to the Dictionary of the Academy, " a patent of invention is given to the author of a new discovery."

Fundamentally, discovery can be logically distinguished from invention, but cannot be separated from it in actual fact. It is often the fertile principle of it ; it causes the new idea to be seen ; invention, which is creative by nature, develops the idea in theory or materializes it as a machine. Hence a new principle is a discovery, but the theory or system derived from it are inventions : the principle of Torricelli concerning the pressure of the atmosphere is a discovery, but all barometers, which are applications of this principle, are inventions. The theory of Branly's coherer is a discovery, while the complete apparatus for wireless telegraphy as constructed by Marconi, is an invention.

However, we need not exaggerate the importance of this distinction. If Poincaré, Laplace, and the majority of engineers habitually confuse inventions and discoveries, they must have serious reasons for doing so. If we examine the question more closely, we find that, in actual fact, there is continual interpenetration between invention and discovery.

[1] Op. cit., p. 128.

In the case of the barometer, the pressure of the air causes the column of mercury to rise to a height of 76 centimetres. Torricelli ascertained a new fact : this was a discovery. But he arrived at it by means of his tube filled with mercury and inverted in a cup of this metal : this was an invention. The discovery and the invention occurred simultaneously.

The same is true of Branly's coherer. The specific action of the filings in cohering under the influence of Herzian waves was a discovery, which was made by means of an invention, namely, the tube of filings with its electrodes. There was a two-fold novelty, both in the principle discovered and in the experiment invented to establish it. Intuitive reason and creative imagination had caught sight of the principle in the light of ·the hypothesis ; the creative imagination, directed by reason, produced the apparatus. We thus have a close alliance between discovery and invention.

That is why, in this inquiry into the rôle of the unconscious in scientific invention, we shall insist before all upon the combinations suggested in inventive constructions by the unconscious factor, but we shall not eliminate its rôle in the discoveries which are the points of departure of the invention. We regard these discoveries as the initial parts of the inventive synthesis, as elements which are distinct from everything but necessary to everything. To study the unconscious in discovery is to examine the passage from night to dawn. But the dawn is the prelude to the full light of day : we shall thus explain the transition from the darkness of night to the full sunshine of invention.

III. SCIENTIFIC INVENTION

We have not, hitherto, attempted to separate by analysis literary or artistic invention from scientific invention. It is time for us to examine the particular characteristics of the latter. The mysterious agent which governs its production, the unconscious, will no doubt operate as it does at the basis of all invention ; but its action will require special conditions, and will take on an original aspect, precisely because the invention is scientific.

It is not without reason that we insist on this distinction. We easily admit the intervention of feeling, and hence of the æsthetic unconscious, in the inspirations of poetic genius and in the conceptions of the artist. For they work in a domain where, at every moment, lively emotion accompanies the austere research of the mind.

But this would not appear to be true of the intuitions of ' the scientist or the creations of the inventor. In their case, we appear to be in the region of facts. Proofs, solid reasons, luminous demonstrations, all these we cannot have too much of : but it is difficult to see what room there is for unconscious sensibility, which is necessarily obscure, in a region entirely exposed to full light.

To this question we shall see that Pascal, Descartes, Henri Poincaré, Ampère and many others reply as follows. The truth newly discovered, the system just invented, the machine constructed, have been desired before being patiently elaborated. This need of a theory or of a new organism preceded its intellectual expression : it existed involuntarily, unconsciously, in the mute aspirations of an individual or a society, before it was clothed in a rational form. Without aiming at it, without understanding why, the creators in the field of science have been unknown artists, in love with a beauty of which they have caught a glimpse, impassioned by a superb ideal. Pasteur, for example, devoted himself to work on crystals before he began his reasearches on microbes. The discoveries of Haüy in crystallography suggested to him the idea of a more general order, that of the great laws of biology. This internal labour was unconscious. We might suppose that no category of knowledge would be farther from feeling than

24 INTRODUCTION

mathematics. Yet Henri Poincaré tells us how great is the importance that he attributes to the feeling for order : " A demonstration is not a simple juxtaposition of syllogisms : the syllogisms are arranged in a certain order, and the order in which the elements are placed is much more important than the elements themselves." The scientist studies Nature " because she is beautiful, not with the beauty of qualities and appearances, but with the more intimate beauty which comes from the harmony of parts, and which pure intelligence can grasp ".[1]

Without anticipating the analyses which form the subject of this study, we may say at once that the place of the unconscious in scientific invention depends precisely upon the rôle of feeling in the sciences.

These inventions are of two kinds ; apparatus, instruments, machines, such as the compass, telescope, rifle, steamship, locomotive. All these may be grouped under the term material inventions. Further, we have theories, systems, new sciences, and so on. These may be called inventions of ideas.

In both cases the psychology of invention is necessarily identically the same : whether it is a matter of combining material elements or associating ideas with a view to a new system, it is always combination that we are dealing with. Hence the mental process followed will always be the same, with its phases of conscious clarity, but also with phases of unconscious elaboration and of subconscious half-shadow.

But since invention is scientific, it will be founded upon previous experience and controlled by further experience, which will form its final verification. Now, as we shall see, the unconscious will enter more especially at two moments : first, in the chance observation which forms the point of departure of the fertile hypothesis, and secondly, in verification, often realized by chance, without previous intention.

[1] Henri Poincaré, *Leçons sur les hypothèses cosmogoniques*, Paris, 1913.

IV. Statement of the Problem and the Method

This preliminary analysis allows us to state clearly the problem to be solved, and to indicate clearly the method to be followed.

To seek the rôle of the unconscious in scientific invention is to determine from the facts what, in various scientific inventions, is conscious, and to distinguish what is in some degree unconscious, and at the same time necessary either as cause or condition. The terms conscious and unconscious will be taken in their widest significance, with all degrees and modalities which we have included in our view.

Hence we shall deal, in the first part, with the domain of the unconscious in knowledge generally, and in the various sciences : mathematics, physics, biology, morals, technology.

We shall then state the results of our inquiry. Everything, whether causes or necessary conditions, which has escaped consciousness, will be classified in the category of unconscious. After this necessary elimination resulting from the facts, we shall pass on to the second part.

In the second part, which deals with the genesis of the invention under the influence of the unconscious, we shall try to explain the psychological elaboration of this inventive work. This will rest entirely upon a theory of integral knowledge, which we shall first develop. Invention will be reduced to intellectual creation, analogous to other mental syntheses.

If it is proved that the unconscious, before all in its dynamic and æsthetic form, has its place and its well defined rôle in judgment, in reasoning, in the various forms of demonstration, it will be natural for it to intervene in the intuitions and combinations of genius. The invention will no longer be an abnormal case, the inventor no longer a kind of thaumaturge. It will be proved that all of us, in various degrees, obey the same psychological laws, and invent to a certain extent. But in the case of the majority, this creative work remains obscure and nameless, because it does not attain a sufficiently high degree. The true invention is a maximum point, the inventor a hero of truth. It will thus afford us satisfaction to have shown that, in the pursuit of progress, good minds may reach the peaks.

FIRST PART

DOMAIN OF THE UNCONSCIOUS IN THE SCIENCES

CHAPTER I

THE UNCONSCIOUS IN KNOWLEDGE IN GENERAL

The unconscious in sensation—In feeling—In perception— In memory—In imagination—In judgment—In reasoning —In our opinions and beliefs—Summary.

KNOWING in every sense of the word is successively *feeling* in some degree, *perceiving, remembering, combining* the ideas received by imagination, *linking* these ideas two by two by the judgment, subjugating the series of judgments by the reason, and finally, as the result of this reasoning, forming opinions on persons and things, the *opinions* being of the nature of rational judgments which have passed to the condition of habits.

In each of these phases of our thought we are brought into contact with the unconscious.

1. *In Sensation*

Sensation consists of two elements : an *affective* element, by which I am agreeably or disagreeably impressed ; and a *significant* element by which I distinguish the particular object which causes me pleasure or pain. I am offered for example a bunch of lilac. I am charmed with its delicate perfume : this is the affective element. But this perfume differs from that of the rose, jasmine, or mignonette ; in this distinctive character I recognize the presence of lilac ; this is the significant element.[1]

Let us analyse this second element. It depends

---

[1] A number of psychologists are wrong in calling it "representative", for it does not represent the nature of the sensation; it is only "the sign of the action of the objects upon the brain". Cf. Dastre: *Revue des Deux Mondes*, April, 1900, p. 680.

necessarily upon previous and similar sensations. In order to attribute to this perfume a known origin, I must have had the same experience in the past in a number of cases. But at the moment when my mind forms the judgment that it is the perfume of lilac, I am in no way thinking of previous judgments. The basis of my affirmation is therefore *unconscious*.

My actual sensation is corroborated by past sensations and is further modified by concomitant present sensations. I drink a sip of Seyssel wine and recognize in this wine the flavour which makes it valuable. A moment after I take a second sip after having eaten some jam, and I find it acid. This change in sensation arises not from the Seyssel wine but from what I have eaten before drinking it.

This difference is caused by the contrast between the sweet taste of the jam and the sharp taste of the wine. However, I have a very clear impression of a change in the sensation. Unknown to me, the change produced by contrast in the effect of the acidity of the wine modified my judgment as to the nature of the liquid. This mental transformation has been *unconscious*.

Numerous facts lead to the same conclusion. Grey in sunshine seems brighter than white in shadow. I look successively at a field coloured in a certain way and at another differently coloured; by contrast the second sensation is relative to the first. I hold a piece of white paper against a white background; then I interpose a piece of coloured paper between the piece of paper and the background: the paper takes the complementary colour.[1]

Thus the actual nature of sensation is not primitive and direct. Reality appears to us under the colours we lend to it. We are accustomed to recognize the colours of objects under various states of daylight, and our mind attributes to them a constant colour without taking account of previous sensations which form the basis of

[1] Leibniz, *Nouveaux essais*, book 11, ch. ix. Cf. Helmholtz, *Physiological optics.*

our judgment. It eliminates in this final judgment the very variable intensity of the light. It even eliminates the colour of the light, and this double elimination is unconscious.

On the other hand, the sensation is not illusory; there really is a sensation present, since we see the object. The idea has produced the corresponding image according to the psychological law of the formation of images.

This mysterious work which is accomplished in sensation had already struck Leibniz. " The ideas which come through sensation," he writes, " are often altered by the mental judgment of the persons experiencing them without their being aware of this fact."

Kant also says the same thing. " To have sense impressions *without being conscious of them,*" he says, " may appear to be a contradiction. How can we know that we have them if we are not conscious of them ? However, we may have · an indirect knowledge of experiencing a sense impression. Kant then gives this example. " I see a man in the distance. I am not conscious of seeing his eyes, his ears, his hands, etc. I see the *man* only. The conclusion is as follows. " The field of obscure sense impression is immense in mankind ; that of conscious impression is very small on the large chart of our mind." [1]

Thus in the immense field of sensations, we find the origin of latent judgments which escape, for the most part, the clear view of our consciousness.

2. *In Feeling*

The generation of the feelings is enveloped in the same obscurity. If, as Wundt thinks, all feeling is in a sense a form of knowledge, we must, for the sake of completeness investigate for a moment the mysterious sources of our affective states. Under *feelings* we understand here all affective states—pleasures or pains—which have a

[1] Kant, *Anthropology*, para. 5.

psychical cause.[1] That is to say, a state of being of the mind, or an idea.

I knew a young man of sixteen who was very depressed, having already failed in his examination for his Batchelor Degree. In his case this prime cause of depression was conscious. But long before his first examination I had found him generally melancholy. This was due no doubt to a number of unfortunate predispositions, of opposing tendencies; perhaps to an inherited hypochondria. In any case the fundamental cause of this mental state was unconscious, as far as the young man was concerned.

This obscure foundation is also found in the origin of joy. Jacques B., my neighbour, is always in a good temper; he is a business man with whom things have gone well for many years. One fine day he exhibits noisy high spirits, which do not surprise anyone, for we know that he has just won five hundred thousand francs at a drawing of the Credit National. When we question him, he tells us of his good luck; the cause of his radiant gaiety is thus quite conscious. But he has never sought for the deep motive of his usual good humour. It is success. It is the fortune he has already built up, it is the attractive qualities which have brought him regular customers. This second cause of his happiness seems to be unconscious.

As well as being the origin of sadness, and the invisible cause of happiness, the unconscious is also the mysterious agent of love. To begin with, we are ignorant of the affection which a person inspires in us. Separation takes place, and the regret which we experience teaches us the true nature of our sentiment. This is a truth which is emphasized by all novelists : Paul and Virginia grew up together, played together, worked together. When they came to the age at which sympathy takes a more active form, they both recognized that they loved one another.

---

[1] We do not say " an idea " as many psychologists seem to require.

Further, as Colsenet remarked, feeling calls up the past and prepares the future. Take a man who is usually gentle. One day, however, exasperated by an opponent, he loses his head and exceeds in a moment the permissible limits of just anger. A latent feeling has awakened in him. It is unconscious atavism. Also, in the secret tendencies about which we do not think there is the promise of a brilliant future. These dispositions, created by hidden feelings, are not all formed : they come into being and are elaborated unconsciously by successive dissociations and associations, from which new combinations result. " This is the origin for us all of desires, of hopes, and of plans ; for a few of us the love of the ideal in the moral life and in Art."[1] This profound thought of Leibniz, " The present is full of the past and pregnant with the future," is true of all our small perceptions and all unconscious feelings.

In the second part of this study, we shall see in what degree feeling is a form of knowledge. For the moment we make our acknowledgment to Wundt, and simply quote his opinion : " In every feeling, in every affection, in every inclination, there is instinctive knowledge. Feeling is even identical with instinctive knowledge, and it appears as soon as knowledge becomes conscious. Feeling only appears in consciousness as a result. It can never recognize a truth ; it can only anticipate it ; it shows the way ; it is the pioneer of knowledge."[2]

Colsenet sums up this doctrine in the passage in which he substitutes tendencies for feelings : " The tendency accompanies the idea which emerges into consciousness. It follows it into unconsciousness and can reappear with it."[3]

We may now ascend a step in the scale of consciousness. Is the unconscious associated with *perception* as well as with sensation and feeling ?

---

[1] Colsenet, op. cit., p. 263.
[2] Cf. Ribot, *La psychologie allemande contemporaine*, p. 265.
[3] Colsenet, op. cit , p. 259.

3. *In Perception*

Reduced to its essential elements, perception is the judgment, implicit or explicit, by which the mind recognizes the existence and qualities of external objects. This intellectual operation i; connected with preceding sensations. To seek the unconscious element of perception is to distinguish in their various phases the various tonalities of attention as far as they are observable, to distinguish the point at which consciousness operates and to separate this instance from the very numerous instances at which consciousness is suppressed.

First of all, the unconscious appears in the three antecedents of perception. (*a*) In its *physical* antecedent, the excitation of the sense organs, which may be slight or often imperceptible, and hence not always reach the threshold of consciousness. (*b*) In its *physiological* antecedent, the impression transmitted to the brain. Some of these impressions are too close to one another to be perceived. (*c*) In its *psychological* antecedent, feeling properly so called, with its two elements, the affective and significant. We have already distinguished, in this double operation, the part which must be played by the unconscious.

Let us proceed at once to the preliminary acts of perception. Various sensations are felt ; they must be distinguished by analysis, and then referred to an external object of a definite nature. First of all, the sensations are projected into space ; we locate them by a primitive and spontaneous judgment of the mind. Why are our visual sensations set out upon a plane perpendicular to the visual axis ? Why, on the other hand, are the nervous impressions communicated to the brain in a different order from those of the parts of the retina ? Because this knowledge of the distribution on the retina is innate, we are told by the nativists ; because this knowledge is acquired, the empiricists reply. How could it be ? Has the mind a second eye for seeing what happens in the first ? On the other hand, the innateness of the nativists explains nothing and is not necessary. The mind may very well distinguish, as Colsenet remarks, the qualitative difference of the sensations given by the elements of the retina, not the position of these elements.[1] Hence the construction of the figure furnished by these elements will be a direct deduction from the sensation. The sensations themselves are conscious ; but their reference to a definite place is made unknown to our minds : it is hence unconscious. Thus the sun appears to us to descend behind the horizon, nevertheless we

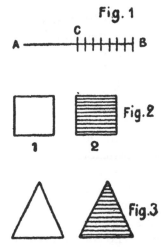

believe the contrary ; in the same way we see behind the plane mirror the reflected virtual image of an object, and yet are aware that it is not there. In this way, the final act from which the synthesis in space of our sensations results is unconscious.

Numerous facts go to show that the formation of the image representing objects is not primitive, and is due to an unconscious process.

Let us mention a few optical illusions.

(1) The straight line AB is divided into two equal parts by the point C ; nevertheless the part CB, which is

1 Colsenet, op. cit., pp. 50–70.

subdivided, appears longer than the part AC which is not subdivided (Fig. 1).

(2) The two squares (1) and (2) are drawn strictly equal in size, but the square (2) which is shaded by parallel lines, appears larger than square (1) which is not so divided (Fig. 2).

(3) The same is true of the equilateral triangles (1) and (2) ; furthermore, in triangle (2) the sides appear longer than the base. These sides are subdivided, while the base is not (Fig. 3).

(4) An empty room appears smaller than a furnished room.

Two explanations have been given for these illusions. Helmholtz says "the perceptible differences appear larger than equal differences which are more difficult to see". According to Dalboeuf, "in the case of the divided line, the duration and number of the muscular efforts made by the eye are greater, hence the time taken is estimated to be longer and hence the space under consideration seems longer also."

This explanation is plausible and explains the judgment of size. But, as there is real perception, that is to say the production of an image, there is therefore real intuition. Now, a simple judgment does not suffice to deal with intuitive appearance. Appeal must be made to the imagination. The idea brings up the image and we attach the same value to both. And as we believe in the reality of the object we also believe in the reality of the image, only, the reasons which have caused the formation of this image are unconscious while the result— the appearance of the image—is conscious.

So far, as regards visual perceptions, we have only considered sensations in a space of two dimensions. We may add the third—depth. Would it be sufficient to make use of the sense of touch to appreciate the distance of objects ? No, for it is necessary to project into space the different points of the object. Would it be said that this projection is an innate faculty ?

But an innate cause would always produce identical effects, while in this case, the conditions and the results of experience vary at every moment. As the processes which bring about this intuitive appearance escape us, and as on the other hand the result is a certain fact, it follows that these processes are unconscious.

It may be said that the distance of the images is proportional to the accommodation of the eye. This is true, but in order to obtain this coefficient of accommodation, it is necessary to bring into play one muscle rather than another with variable intensity. We are absolutely ignorant of what determines this coefficient or degree of intensity.

Passing from perceptions of sight to those of hearing, we are in no way more enlightened as to the movements of the larynx necessary for the production of a certain note. We do not make any conscious calculation, and nevertheless we attack the note with remarkable accuracy. To say that it is the result of habit is to refuse to face the problem, for as regards habit it is necessary to find out whether the phenomenon is conscious or unconscious. In this case it is certainly unconscious.

The unconscious is thus largely represented in the preliminary operation of perception, and we may ask whether it plays a part in the actual act of perception, which is knowledge. More precisely, is there an unconscious element in the mental act by which the intuitive or auditive appearance is referred to a general idea which determines it ?

" A hat and an overcoat characterize a man," says Descartes. Is this affirmation a judgment or even a piece of unconscious reasoning ? Many people have maintained that it is. Colsenet does not think so : " Habit and association suffice to explain how our mind is presented with the general idea called up by certain sensible qualities to which we have previously united it." [1]

Does this solve the problem ? If habit and association

[1] Op. cit., p 96.

have, in the past, united certain sensible qualities to form a general idea, the combination was certainly quite conscious at the time of its formation, but is it so now ? The result appears conscious, but the complex of ideas which previously justified the judgment of perception is actually unconscious. In making this positive statement, the mind is in possession of the results of a past conscious state, but at the moment when it makes its statement, its motives are unconscious. In making this examination of the part played by perception, we shall pass over various much discussed theories of perception, such, for instance, as assimilation (Aristotle and the Scholastics), intuitive perception (Hamilton and Garnier), atomistic emission (Democritus), sensorial impressions (Maine de Biran), representative ideas (Locke), ideas produced by God in us (Berkeley), intuition of divine ideas (Malebranche), immediate suggestion (Reid), true hallucination (Stuart Mill and Taine). We shall pause at the theory of inference maintained by Descartes and Cousin. This is based upon rational interpretation, and hence should, if not suppress, at least reduce to a minimum the part played by the unconscious.

We arrive at the knowledge of an external object by means of two principles, those of *causality* and of *substance*. I see an apple. I immediately recognize by the principle of causality that the cause of this sensation is external to myself. The effect, sensation, is real, hence the external cause must be real also. It is determined by the collaboration of all my senses ; sight gives me the colour, smell the odour, taste the savour, touch the resistance, form, temperature, etc. At this point, the principle of substance allows me to unify these coexistent sensations ; a single subject, the apple, furnishes the *substratum* of these various phenomena of sense. Hence I know that the object is an apple.

The animal which recognizes its master, the child which distinguishes its mother, and the adult in most circumstances of his life, do not perform this process of reasoning. It may be performed by the medical expert engaged on a legal problem, the archæologists who, by means of various signs carefully discussed, recognize an ancient monument, the geologist who discovers a fossil, and by certain other specialists. Habitually, however, we affirm the existence of external objects without interpreting the sensations produced by these objects, by our instinct alone. Hence the judgment and reasoning necessary in certain cases and always possible, are most often taken for granted. We are fully conscious in affirm:ng the existence of such objects ; but the causal nexus which justifies our certainty at any moment, is certainly unconscious at the precise moment of perception, although it may have been conscious in the past.

4. *In Memory*

A considerable part of the phenomena of perception which are transitory by nature, is preserved in memory. We must therefore investigate the part played by the unconscious in our recollection.

How are we to explain the preservation of our recollection ? By the vibratory movement of nerve fibres ? But this movement was only a condition for the registration of ideas. It is necessary to explain the possibility of the recollection of these ideas.

If the vibrations begin with the idea, and then disappear when the idea leaves our consciousness and finally are renewed at the moment of recollection, how do we recognize the second series of vibrations as being like the first, if the first disappears entirely ?

If the vibrations begun in the organism at the moment of the inception of the idea are prolonged in some fashion, they must prolong in some way the psychical fact ; the second series of vibrations, similar to the first, recall the psychical fact and distinguish it from perception or from a fact of the imagination. In this case, there would be true recollection. This necessary hypothesis is thus true. Recollection " is an application of intellectual activity to the reproduction of an idea previously conceived. It is a case of habit. All being tends to continue to exist ; thus ideas are rethought as originally thought, the more easily because we react them in making them our own, by virtue of the tendency of our mind to activity ".[1]

But this habit is not a " bare and undetermined " activity. As Leibniz said : *Quod non agit, non existit.* Thus an activity, the act of which is the idea, must also be determined by an idea which is at least begun. This means that there remains in us, as the foundation of our memories, the elementary act which constitutes the future idea, the idea in the inchoate state. What remains in our memory is more than an aptitude. It is a psychological fact, the germ of an idea, corresponding to an organic fact. But this is not the complete idea as it will reappear in consciousness. It will appear enlarged and developed.

This is a little like Stuart Mill's thought, in his refutation of Hamilton : " What is latent is not the latent impressions, but the power of reproducing them.[2]

Thus, stated more precisely, what is preserved in memory is, in the organism, a vibratory movement or the form of a transmitted wave, and in the mind, a sensation or the germ of an idea.[3]

But this ferment of memory does not appear in consciousness. Bouillier, from whom we have borrowed the preceding analysis, is guilty of a confusion of terms when he concludes " there is no such thing as the unconscious ; forgetting is the persistence of ideas

---

[1] Gratcap, *Thèse sur la memoire*, Paris ; cf. Colsenet, op. cit., pp. 222–4.
[2] S. Mill, *Examination of the Philosophy of Hamilton.*
[3] Bouillier, *La principe vitale et l'âme pensante*, ch. xxii, p. 405.

externally to my own consciousness ". As we call unconscious to some extent all that escapes actual consciousness, we may simply say that this preservation of memory is unconscious : unconscious in the association of ideas which can call it up and which has served to fix the recollection, for the point of attachment is often unknown ; unconscious in the obscure tendencies which have made it easy ; unconscious finally and above all, in the crop of ideas which come to us at every instant, and which expand on a mass of memories about which we do not think. This latent persistence of the immense number of ideas received in the past is attested by a number of philosophers in many interesting ways.

" Thought is one thing," says Plotinus, " the perception of our thought another . . . We are always thinking, but we do not always preceive our thoughts." [1]

St. Augustine, long before Leibniz, propounded a theory of the unconscious in memory. He admits the difference between knowing a thing and thinking of it, and he thus characterizes unconscious mental phenomena, which he distinguishes from conscious phenomena : " Ideas do not emerge from the mind ; they are there without our knowing it. Learning is nothing else than grouping ideas in such a way that they are, as it were, ready to hand and come to us at the first sign. Thinking consists in reassembling the ideas scattered and dispersed in memory, and perhaps in bringing them back to the unity of consciousness." [2] Elsewhere, he thus shows that the domain of the unconscious borders on that of consciousness : " I do not know myself all that I am."

Leibniz enlarges this doctrine. He distinguishes apperception, clearly and distinct conscious, from perception, which is an internal state of the monad and represents external things. Perceptions are more or less confused. Minor perceptions are unconscious.

---

[1] Enneads, 4, lib. iii, 30.
[2] *Confessions*, lx, ch. ii. Cf. Ferraz, *La psychologie de Saint Augustin,* 1862 ; Nourrisson, *La philosophie de Saint Augustin,* 1865.

Memory, and the knowledge of necessary truths, are the conditions for apperception or clear consciousness. But since this apperception " has not been given to all minds nor even at all times to the same mind, phases of obscurity and unconsciousness exist in every mind ". This mysterious domain is very large : " For a monad only knows a part of its perfections, otherwise every monad would be a divinity." On the other hand the soul or monad is a perpetual living mirror of the Universe. Hence an infinity of perceptions must escape it. Such perceptions are those obscure ones which are deficient only in respect of the capability for being recollected, and which, in every substance, " keep the future in perfect contact with the past." [1]

Kant also, in a chapter on unconscious representation, exposes to our view the immensity of the field occupied by the unconscious in memory : " A superior power would only have to say ' Let there be light ! ' (if for example we take a literary man with all his recollections) to call up without any addition the half of a world to his eyes." [2]

Hartmann, of course, who made so much use of the unconscious has also charged it with the duty of elaborating memories. Thus in linking the theory of memory to the rest of his system, he expresses himself as follows : " Every idea is new. If a memory is recognized in it it is because the idea is formed for the first time in the bosom of the *unconscious*. Memories are formed like feeble echoes of the preceding perceptions." [3]

This rôle of memory in the formation of ideas is recognized by Dwelshauvers, whom we have already had occasion to quote. The unconscious reserves form the inexhaustible soil upon which new ideas grow at every instant, all of them so many inventions in miniature.

---

[1] *Principes de la Nature et de la Grace fondés en raison*, Dutens Edition, vol. ii, p. 33.
[2] Kant, *Anthropologie*, par. 5.
[3] *Philosophie de l'inconscient*, vol. i, pp. 337–40.

5. *In Imagination*

Let us first distinguish the imagination from the imaginative memory, which reproduces the idea and the image left by a perception in the memory. The imagination on the other hand transforms the representations acquired into new syntheses ; it disassociates groups formed by the memory in order to utilize their elements in new combinations ; ideas, perceptions, feelings, are all materials which may enter into a construction formed by the imagination.

It is evident that the result of these combinations is conscious. The poems of a writer, the pictures of a painter, the machines of an inventor, the theory of a sociologist, are ends attained by their creators, who are conscious of them.

But the long work of incubation which has preceded the appearance of the masterpiece carries many traces of the unconscious. We may convince ourselves of this by examining imaginative work in its three principal forms : reverie, dream, and ordinary meditation.

In reverie, the intelligence is not directed by the will ; it passes from one association to the other ; groups of ideas are presented to the view of the consciousness, like the movable faces of a rose-window. The result is conscious, the elaborate process by which it has been prepared, is not so.

The part mysteriously hidden is still larger in the case of the *dream*. Here there is no reflection, no voluntary direction. Disassociations and associations are formed solely according to the psychological law of the production of images. They are unconscious.

In the case of *meditation* we have the collaboration of will and reflection. Here also the unconscious certainly plays a part, for, although the subject under investigation is clearly present in the mind's eye, this is not true of the various phases of the meditation. Ideas hatch out suddenly. Why one particular one rather than another ?

Conceptions arise, doubtless linked with the general idea, but capable of replacement by others equally logical. Why should some appear rather than others ? Their formation has been unconscious. Examples are numerous. For instance, we seek in vain the solution of a geometrical problem. At the moment when we give up thinking about it, the correct figure appears quite suddenly to our imagination. Thus the result alone is known.

But although the greater part of the work of meditation is unconscious, our will has a part to play. This consists, not in actually arousing the production of ideas, but in setting certain conditions which, when brought together, are favourable to the particular kind of conception which is desired. We may examine this more closely.

The ruling idea appears and is conscious ; the inventor, for example, is clearly aware that he has in view the construction of a machine. But this requires long-continued effort ; the will keeps the idea in consciousness. It forms a point of departure.

Immediately, in view of the solution proposed, combinations rise into the mind.` How are they formed ? Why some and not others ? We do not know ; the operation is quite *unconscious*. Then, in the service of the intellect, the will eliminates one hypothesis and retains another. It is guided in this conscious selection by a more general idea, the formation of which has been *unconscious*. This idea intervenes in the various judgments.

Finally, the right idea is found. One association rather than another has been forced to appear ; the absence of sensation has facilitated the discovery during the night or early in the morning. The mind being freer is more active and sure. The result appears suddenly to consciousness.

We see that the associations have been formed in secret in the unconscious. But the elements of which they are composed have passed through consciousness. This is why in a sense discoveries and inventions are prepared by long and methodical work. Hartmann himself recognizes this fact : " The inspired idea appears even if other parts of the brain are occupied by altogether different thoughts, provided that an association of ideas, however weak it may be, gives the impulse to the causality of the unconscious." Thus the unconscious does not work alone. It needs favourable ground, that is to say, a mind full of ideas and appropriate images.

There is no need, however, to look for a mysterious *deus* in this work of fertile transformation. At this point we diverge from Hartmann and say with Leibniz : " It is the mind which is the creator ; the soul is an image of the Divinity ; it is creative in its voluntary act and, in discovering the sciences, it imitates in its department, and in the small world where it is allowed to operate, what God does in the great world."

Goethe, a few days before his death, distinguished as follows the moments of obscure generation and the phases of pure clarity in the synthetic work of the mind :

" Every power to act and hence every talent implies an instinctive force acting in the unconscious in ignorance of rules, the principle of which is none the less present. The sooner a man educates himself, the sooner he learns that he has a calling, an art which will furnish him the means of obtaining the full development of his natural faculties, the more fortunate he is. What comes to him from outside, what he acquires, can never injure in the slightest degree his individuality. The highest genius is that which assimilates everything and can appropriate everything without injury to its innate character. Here we come across the various connections between consciousness and the unconscious. The organs of a man, by the work of exercise, of apprenticeship, of persistent and continuous reflection, by movements of appeal and resistance, these organs amalgamate and combine unconsciously what is instinctive and what is acquired. From this amalgamation, from this combination, from this chemistry at once conscious and unconscious, there finally results an harmonious whole which excites the wonder of the world." [1]

6. In Judgment

The judgment we are concerned with here is not the faculty of separating the true from the false, but the operation of the mind which perceives and affirms the agreement between two ideas. It is made up of three elements : the two ideas brought into connection and the affirmation of this connection. It will be *analytical* if it is a simple decomposition of the subject into its constituent elements, and synthetic if, as a result of experience, the attribute is added to the subject. This distinction will suffice for the question we are concerned with.

If we are to believe Hartmann, " Every particular idea may receive in its comprehension a large number of general ideas . . . Otherwise expressed, the subject may contain attributes. In fact, its receives the attributes corresponding to the end in view." Let us examine his position more closely. Take the judgment : snow is white. The subject snow may evidently receive other qualifiers, expressing its attributes. I may say the snow is cold, the snow is melting, etc. Why did I stop at its whiteness ? The reason may be that I am a painter, a poet, or simply a natural admirer of the external aspect of things. By means of my judgment I have made a choice among *n* possible attributes, but this choice has been instinctive, hence unconscious. It corresponds to my psychical disposition. What is unconscious is not the actual act of affirmation. In saying that the snow is white, I am clearly aware of what I am stating ; but I, do not think at all of the invisible state of my mind at the moment, or my psychical antecedents.

[1] Letter to W. von Humboldt, 17th March, 1832.

7. *In Reason*

Here, side by side with the clarity of conscious logic, we can distinguish fringes of unconsciousness. Hartmann finds that they play a large part. He starts from the actual mechanism of thought. " Thinking," he says, " is analysing, uniting, or co-ordinating. We abstract and unite in a single notion *n* simple ideas. This notion only contains the common element. This common element is suddenly presented to the mind by inspiration. Reasoning is performed by combination. We have an idea, we seek another ; it is furnished by the unconscious. In the syllogism the minor and the conclusion are conscious ; but a suitable major is chosen which frequently remains unconscious. Hence the general premise need not present itself to my thought. The conclusion alone appears in consciousness." [1]

After this general theory of reasoning, Hartmann discusses some of its forms. " In induction, the understanding gets back instinctively to the cause by the unconscious logic of the mind. In mathematics, intuitive logic tells us without demonstration that the three angles of an equilateral triangle are equal. In higher mathematics, mathematicians suppress long series by rapid intuition. Still more intimate communion with the *unconscious* would reveal everything by intuition." [2]

Elsewhere, he adopts the following reflections of Jessen. " We reflect about an object, then we think of something else ; our activity is pursued unconsciously. When we return to the subject, a kind of revelation is made to us : the result of thought is presented clearly to consciousness. Sometimes we make great efforts without finding any ideas. Quite suddenly, some time afterwards, a flood of ideas pours in." [3]

[1] Op. cit., pp. 335, 337, 340, 241, 343.
[2] Op. cit., p. 348.
[3] Jessen, *Psychologie*, p. 235, 236 ; quoted by Hartmann, op. cit., vol. i, p. 353.

Hartmann, following Schopenhauer, shows clearly how a change of opinion is produced in us as the result of a lecture or discussion.

" We read a book, we reject an opinion without refuting it. Then we forget it. Later we return to it, and the opinion appears correct to us. Our thoughts have ruminated unconsciously, then digested and assimilated." [1]

Joseph Jastrow says almost the same thing in his work on the subconscious :—

" In every effort which is made in the intellectual field, there is a period of incubation, a process for the most part subconscious, a slow and hidden development accompanied by the absorption of appropriate nutriment. This is what Schopenhauer calls " unconscious rumination ". A rumination of our thoughts which prepares them for assimilation by our mental tissues. We are thus able to formulate two principles, which are nothing but two abstracts of the same thesis. The first of these principles is that the process of assimilation can take place even when conscious activity is very much reduced ; the second is that most of the influences which determine our mental development may be effective without acting directly in the light of our conscious life." [2]

These phases of unconsciousness in the evolution of thought are not admitted by Desdouits :—

" When the wise man," he says, " divines a truth by intuition, is it true that he thinks unconsciously of all the logical intermediate steps ? This is a useless hypothesis, for these apparent divinations, these almost direct conclusions can be explained quite naturally by known laws. The mind thinks by analogy, or by passing rapidly through the intermediate steps, or by some of these steps and the law which governs them, but consciousness is always present. Divination by

---

[1] Hartmann, op. cit., p. 355.
[2] Jastrow, op. cit., p. 69.

analogy is common among inventors ; it is almost always the analogy between the imagined law and known laws which has put the scientist on his way to the hypothesis. Or sometimes the rapidity is explained by habit ; the mind jumps over the intermediate steps."

This explanation by analogy and habit of the mystery which surrounds reasoning not completely formulated, does not solve the problem. For, in analogy and habit we again find the unconscious, to some extent at least.

To appreciate at their true value these various opinions, we may run through the different forms of reasoning, and consider in each case where consciousness stops and the unconscious commences.

In the first place, is the syllogism with its three formal propositions fully conscious ? Hartmann is right in questioning this. The conclusion is plainly conscious ; the minor which prepares the conclusion and which follows from the major is also conceived in full clarity. But as regards the major, we may ask why is one taken rather than another. Because one responds to the question under debate, because it is a principle which may be made use of in the following discussions. Because it is a means of obtaining a logical end, the conclusion to be established. If it is the commencement of a solution, others were possible. If it is a principle, others might have been applied equally well. If it is a means, it is generally not the only means. Why this particular commencement, this particular principle, this particular means, in preference to others ?

Because this logical result has been prepared by antecedent thoughts which had been forgotten, suggested by latent preoccupation, formed by past meditation or reading without our knowledge. This more distant origin of the syllogism is unconscious.

Is it true, as Hartmann thinks, that in irregular syllogisms, the unconscious maintains its activity as

----

¹ Desdouits, op. cit., pp. 74–6.

E

regards premises which are taken for granted ? There are many distinctions to be made. In the enthymeme, the argument is reduced to two propositions, or even to one. But the premises which are not expressed are thought by a rapid intuition ; the consciousness plays in this case a fugitive and partial rôle ; but this prevents our having to deal with the purely unconscious.

The same observation may be made concerning the polysyllogism and the sorites ; the propositions are joined : those which are not explicitly formulated are only in part unconscious. The epichirema with its premises accompanied by their proof, offers for the unconscious a field as much reduced as possible. It has no place when once reasoning has begun ; it can only play a part as in the case of the regular syllogism in the preliminary incubation from which the fertile major proceeds.

In the operation of induction we start from the facts and seek for the law, we ascend from the conditioned to the condition, from the effect to its cause. This is done by observation, and by experiment, which is observation under prepared conditions. In these two operations, which require attention and reflection, everything is conscious excepting for the very small part of sensation and perception absorbed by the unconscious.

But after a few observations we find that an hypothesis is conceived. This is an anticipation of the law, and an idea which directs further research. It is apparently a sudden vision, a flash of genius. As a product of the creative imagination, it formulates an imagined law, a law without proof. Half glimpsed as a possibility, it is " the distant princess " which pleases the imagination without yet satisfying the reason. Whence does it come ? Is it the result of conscious deduction ? It would be rash to make such an assumption ; on the contrary all scientists recognize the suddenness of its appearance. It is the golden star which leads the wise man to the truth, without his knowing whence the brilliant meteor comes.

Nevertheless it has a psychical cause. Newton saw an apple fall to the ground, and soon afterwards thought of universal gravitation. Universal gravitation was the hypothesis ; the fall of the apple was the fact observed. How did he pass from one to the other ? By a kind of latent reasoning of the following kind : This apple falls, other bodies have already fallen, others will fall. The order of the world is constant ; hence there is a general law which produces the fall of bodies. Thus the hypothesis was conceived.

Fundamentally, it is a uniformity which is conceived as the result of many similar observations, hence it is formed by way of resemblance or analogy. We are thus brought to consider what traces of the unconscious' are to be found in reasoning by analogy.

This consists in deducing from an observed resemblance an invisible resemblance. For example, from the fact that the sense organs are similar in man and animal, we deduce that their sensations are likewise similar.

The mechanism of this kind of reasoning consists in passing from the particular to the particular by way of a general idea. Logically considered, it includes an induction followed by a deduction. I see, for example, in A the elements ab associated to produce c. On the other hand, I find again in B the elements ab. By means of an induction I can understand and formulate this law. ab followed by c in A will always be followed by c in similar associations. I then draw this deduction : ab have always produced c ; they will therefore produce it in B.

But in order to reason in this way without obvious sophism, I must without thinking about it be guided by a latent principle, one which is very general and very fertile, and which might be formulated as follows : *the universe, in spite of the diversity of its constituent parts, is made up of many similar plans, which explain one another. The world of ideas, the moral world, and the sensible world are expressions in different terms of the same thought.*

This is, in another form, the double principle of indiscernables and of continuity put forward by Leibniz, the first explaining the diversity, the second rendering plausible the general similarity of the elements of the Cosmos. The monad of Leibniz which reflects the entire universe, is the world of Plato and the Alexandrines, the gigantic animal which gives life to a single breath expressed in different form.

From this fundamental premise unconsciously impressed upon my mind, I can deduce all the rich litany of literary, scientific, or philosophical analogies. In this way a great initial analogy suggests numerous derived ones. This is the unconscious phase. The analogies are formulated more precisely, and take the form of anticipated laws or hypotheses, and these, as the ideas directing scientific work, suggest experiment and verification from which scientific laws are derived. This is the conscious phase.

8. *In our Opinions and Beliefs*

If we now leave the more fully characterized forms of reasoning and seek the origin of our opinions, our beliefs, and our doubts, we find with Hartmann that " the most deeply rooted opinions are the result of an unconscious process ". What is not done by conscious reasoning is done by the unconscious ; for conscious reasoning is critical, it sifts ideas and submits them to severe control. On the other hand, the unconscious is subjected to the influence of interests and leanings. The synthesis formed in its depths is made of richer and more varied elements. It is in this mysterious way that there are formed at a given moment, concerning men and things, completed judgments, deep seated opinions which often reach impregnable certainty. What is the origin of these sudden changes of mind, these conversions of soul ? The factors are doubtless numerous ; heriditary tendency going far back into the past, education, the profound effect of reading or discussion or of a disturbing word heard by chance, often the charm of a close friendship. On analysis, the psychologists find conscious traces of certain of these causes. They form a track similar to that left in the sky by the medley of clouds called cirro-cumulus. But these relics of past thought are not sufficient to explain the present existence of the firm opinion. Unconscious elements must have played a part in the mental synthesis, but their traces have been lost.

For this mental synthesis is always operating, incorporating appropriate elements, unifying our intellectual acquisitions, and sometimes modifying them in the melting pot of its unconscious logic. In every rational operation, the unconscious plays a part. The mind becomes like a sea which is always agitated ; at every moment an unknown wave arises from its mysterious depth and cuts across the superficial wave. My actual conscious thought—doubt, belief, or certainty—is the sparkling sunlit surface which results in the interferences of the unconscious psychical waves.

9. Summary

The analysis of the various phases of knowledge in general has led us to the following result.

The unconscious appears in the significant element, or in the latent judgment which allows us to appreciate our sensations ; it explains habitual sadness, good humour, the progressive evolution of love, and all other feelings ; it gives an account of illusions in optics, of judgments of size and harmony, which are isolated in our perception the judgment itself of which escapes us ; it is the germ of the idea which precedes the appearance of a recollection from our memory. In imaginative work, it causes the elaboration of the reverie and the dream and the production of various ideas as a result of meditation. It reappears in the judgment, which is the conclusion of a latent operation of thought. Here it is that the slow rumination takes place from which comes the majors of syllogisms, the formation of hypotheses in induction, and general analyses which prepare hypotheses or derived analogies. Finally, by its action on our sensibility, the unconscious produces our opinions, our beliefs, our doubts ; it is the mysterious agent which at the end of a long period of obscure or semi-obscure incubation, produces a mental synthesis.

But these sensations, these feelings, these perceptions, these products of memory and these constructions of the imagination, these judgments and these reasonings, all these opinions with their various degrees of certainty can be found in all thinking. In fact, all thought is an intellectual operation ; on the other hand all thought differs from what has preceded it and also from what will follow it. All thought is thus something new, is an invention, consequently, in view of the preceding analysis, the various scientific inventions considered simply as thoughts and systems of thought will present us in their formation with an ample supply of unconscious elements.

We may go further. All invention is combination. Hence scientific inventions are combinations of scientific elements. Now these combinations are various ; on the other hand, the elements constituting these inventions are furnished by methods which are as various as the nature of the elements themselves. The co-operation of feeling and reason, of the unconscious and the consciousness, is truly present in all these inventions since they are all systems of thought, but will take on a specific character from one science to another. It is our task to investigate to what degree and in what form the unconscious and the consciousness play a part in various scientific inventions.

We will commence with mathematics.

Chapter II

THE UNCONSCIOUS IN MATHEMATICAL INVENTION

The opinion of theorists—Descartes and Analytical Geometry—Pascal and his mathematical invention—Leibniz and Newton, the Infinitismal Calculus—Monge and Descriptive Geometry—Laplace—Ampère and Gauss—Inaudi—Henri Poincaré—E. Faguet—A personal experience—Summary.

A CCORDING to M. Thomas, the object of the mathematical sciences is to determine the properties of numbers and of figures defined in space, and the laws of correlative variations between different magnitudes.[1]

I. *The Opinion of Theorists : Descartes, Leibniz, A. Comte, Laisant*

The foregoing remark is very well put. But for our purpose, we may follow Descartes, and connect mathematical concepts with the two ideas of *order* and *measurement* : " The more carefully I have considered these matters," he says, " the more clearly have I recognized that the only ideas to be brought into mathematics are those of order and measurement." [2]

Leibniz simplifies this still further : " Measurement only exists," he thinks, " where order previously existed." [3]

The inventor of the Infinitesimal Calculus is right. Measuring consists in expressing a relation between a quantity or a magnitude and a unit of the same nature. But before defining this relation, the terms of it must be conceived ; that is to say, a relation based upon the identity of the parts constituting a whole must be

---

[1] *Cours de philosophie*, p. 268.
[2] Ibid., author's note.
[3] Op. cit. et loc. cit., author's note.

thought. Hence, this whole must have been distinguished from others : prior to the calculation, a mental classification of measurable objects must have taken place. Consequently, two of these objects, one being the unit contained n times in the other which is to be measured, have been arranged in the same series by a previous act of identification. Thus it is the idea of order which is fundamental in mathematics ; it will suggest all hypotheses ; it will direct the whole work of invention in this field.

But this idea, which is a general postulate in all demonstrations, has been taken for granted by every algebrician and geometer. We ourselves, following Leibniz and Descartes, have been obliged, in order to bring it to light, to perform a process of analysis. This amounts to saying that this fundamental basis of the exact sciences is unconscious. Thus, before we invoke the testimony and experience of mathematicians, it is important to note that this conclusion is rational.

Auguste Comte realized this fact. In defining the means for the development of the sciences—and we know that by this he meant chiefly mathematics—he says : " The progress of any science consists alternately in the perfection of the technical part or technique, and of the method." [1]

Now method is only order in the pursuit of truth. It is right application of the mind ; for, as Descartes says, " It is not enough to have a good mind ; the essential thing is to apply it rightly."

That is why the great builders of mathematics, Descartes, Pascal, Newton, Cauchy, Poincaré, etc., have been men of method.

To this first unconscious source, order, we may suitably add the investigatory procedure which governs all scientific experiment. Doubtless, as Laisant, following Poincaré, observes : " In mathematics, only a minimum

---

[1] Comte, *Essai sur la philosophie des mathématiques*, Paris.

of notions is borrowed from experience." But these authors add at once : " All science is experimental." [1]

It was by experiment that the following properties were discovered : the relation between the circumference and diameter of a circle is nearly equal to $\frac{16}{9}$; triangles having sides in the proportion 3 : 4 : 5 are right-angled ; the sum of consecutive odd numbers, starting with 1, is always a perfect square ; and so on. But in these experiments, there existed the obscure phases which we have pointed out in sensations and perceptions. Hence, under this aspect alone, mathematics already contains a considerable element of the unconscious. [2]

2. *Descartes and Analytical Geometry*

This element is much larger if we examine the part played by the *imagination* in the exact sciences. Laisant, in the work just quoted, thus explains the origin of our geometrical notions : " We observe the regularity of objects, and their form. These regular arrangements assume an existence in our brain by *unconscious* abstraction. [3]

. But, long before Laisant, Descartes had defined this rôle of the imagination in this representation of mathematical notions :—

" The idea," he writes in his *Regulae*, " is the work of God, who created it immutable and eternal. Imagination intervenes to perfect sensible images. The imagination will be a means of verification. But by itself, it would be a cause of error ; it must co-operate with the understanding. Thus the image will be the immediate cause which makes the idea pass from the power to the act. On the other hand, the imagination makes us see the changeable side of things : it gives us an incomplete

---

[1] Laisant, *La Mathématique*, Paris, 1898.

[2] Cf. Comte, *Cours de philosophie positive*, III lecon. Salande, *Lectures sur la philosophie des sciences*, Ch. III.

[3] Laisant, op. cit., p. 90.

knowledge. But once fixed on an object, it does not lose its way : as a result, it serves to awaken in us certain ideas. Its part will be played chiefly in geometry, but even in algebra. It is necessary to exclude from algebra every notion which is not susceptible of being represented by an image." [1]

We know how Descartes put into practice these principles in dealing with the part played by the imagina-

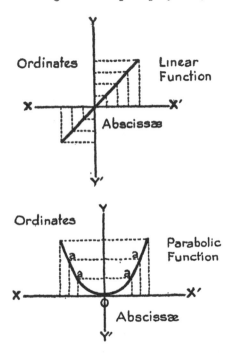

tion. He was the inventor of analytical geometry, which embodied his theory of the co-ordinates now called Cartesian. By using two rectangular axes, the one horizontal and representing the value of the variable x or t, the other vertical and representing the value of the function y, the author shows that the equation $y = ax$ is represented by a straight line passing through the meeting point O of the two axes. In the same way he

[1] Descartes, *Regulae*, xii, 80.

expresses the equation $y = ax^2$ by a parabola, the symmetrical points of which are a_1 and a_2, a_3 and a_4, etc. Other functions are dealt with in the same way. It is not a matter for us in this psychological study to set out tables of variations and to justify the exactness of these representative figures. These proofs are to be found in the textbooks of elementary algebra. Our intention is to couple this invention with the author's theory concerning the imagination, and to distinguish in it the unconscious and the conscious. What origin must we assign to this theory of developed functions, as stated by Descartes, Legendre, Cauchy and Jacobi? Is it sufficient to invoke, as Laisant does, the fact of the double periodicity of functions? [1]

It is true that $f(x)$ takes on similar values for the different values of x. But it is necessary first of all to note this similarity in the results : before noting it, it was necessary to make calculations which showed this uniformity. It is true that Descartes does not tell us what chance circumstance led him to this result. But his principles reveal the internal mechanism of his thought : he wished to verify a theory by means of its expression in images. This theory was still in an embryonic state. The experiment succeeded ; the representation produced by the imagination formed a confirmation. This is why he writes : " The image is the immediate cause which makes the idea pass from potentiality to activity." In the whole of his theory, functions exist potentially previous to experience. This is the partially unconscious phase. Subsequently, the attempts at representation, when they have fully succeeded, " have served to awake in him certain ideas " ; the theory is completed on definite lines in full consciousness. The original point of this doctrine, is as we have seen, the substitution of an image for an algebraic formula, and we have established in the preceding chapter, that every creation of an image by the imagination is unconscious.

[1] Laisant, op. cit., p. 88.

3. *Pascal and his Mathematical Inventions*

If now we turn from Descartes to Pascal, we first of all discover methods of work interesting to note in connection with unconscious invention. Descartes was above all a strict observer of method. His *Discours* and his *Quatre règles* are sufficient to point out his mental disposition in this respect. Pascal follows, apparently, the opposite path. In his feverish desire to make discoveries, he passes from one idea to another, and bears with difficulty the onerous yoke of intellectual discipline. Consequently he cannot force himself to pursue for long on end the solution of a given problem, excepting only in the construction of the calculating machine at which he worked for nine years.

We may note this discontinuity in his researches, these variations in the objectives, and this relatively unforeseen nature of the results.

Let us take a few of these results. As regards his reconstitution of Euclid's *Elements of Geometry*, it has been claimed that Pascal was acquainted with them. His work would thus not have been an invention, but the reconstitution of learned principles made by a highly gifted mind. If we admit this point of view, we must at least recognize that this reconstitution was unconscious ; for Pascal nowhere speaks of the sources which inspired it, and on the other hand, criticism should not go to the length of suspecting the good faith of a person otherwise so straightforward and sincere.

But since there is a dispute on this point, we will only attach a relative importance to this discovery, and see whether we cannot find traces of the unconscious in his other mathematical inventions.

There is nothing of especial note in his *Essay on Conic Sections*, written at the age of sixteen, utilizing the researches of Desargeus, the mathematician of Lyons. Everything appears also quite conscious in his treatise on the *Arithmetical Triangle* : a succession of whole numbers arranged in vertical columns forms a triangle ; each number is formed by taking the sum of those above it. All the more, before the elaboration of the theory, we must imagine his surprise at obtaining an unexpected result by trial and error, a surprise which must have incited the investigator to develop his proof.

But in the origin of his work on the *Calculus of Probabilities*, on the *Cycloid*, and on the calculating machine, there was present an ardent desire with all the unconscious elements which form its psychical support. It was in order to answer two questions put to him by the Chevalier de Mère that Pascal found an equation of finite differences, and applied to the Calculus of Probablities the theory of combinations recently invented by Fermat. It was a challenge thrown down to mathematicians which stimulated him to solve the problem of the Cycloid, with the theory of summations and integrations. Finally it was with the object of being useful to his father that he conceived at Rouen the first idea of the calculating machine known by his name. This machine only performs addition and subtraction. The idea was also not new, for Leibniz, at about the same time, had sketched the construction of a machine giving the result of all operations. Pascal was the first who carried out partially this idea.[1]

Thus in these three cases, invention was stimulated by desire ; feeling produced research. But we have seen, in the first chapter, what is implied by feeling in potential intellectual operations. Pascal was a striking example of the unconscious power of desire in the service of invention.

4. *Leibniz, Newton, and the Infinitèsimal Calculus*

A similar stimulus urged two geniuses, at about the same time, Leibniz and Newton, to the invention of the

[1] Picard (E.), *Pascal, Mathematicien et physicien*, Paris, 1923, pp. 1–12.

infinitesimal calculus. In order to realize the importance of the problem to be solved, and the nature of the intellectual operations, conscious or unconscious, which governed them in this common aim, let us state the question in debate in a few words.

Algebraic notation accurately expresses the continuity of the variations of x and y, but only from one interval to another, for these symbols are numbers, and hence terms representing discontinuity. When these algebraic methods are applied to the study of accelerated or retarded movement, they prove insufficient. The choice of sufficiently small units, it is true, allows us to arrive at closer and closer approximations, but never at continuity. It is necessary, therefore, to introduce into the calculation infinitely small increments, smaller than any given quantity. Although infinitely small, they will have the properties of given quantities, but being smaller than any given quantity they will never be one. But they are introduced in order to obtain continuity, and this is the object of the *differential calculus*. Finally, in order to return to whole quantities susceptible of numerical interpretation, they are eliminated by the *integral calculus*.[1] In Leibniz's case, this search for mathematical continuity is only an aspect of his doctrine of universal continuity. On the other hand, the infinitely small quantities which he makes use of in his calculation recall the infinitely numerous monads whose analogous constitution and progressive perfection form the harmonious unity of the Universe. Thus in the mental synthesis taking place in this extraordinary mind, the new calculus, which he ardently desired in order to satisfy his philosophical system, was sketched in successive stages, partly conscious, since they contained long meditated logical developments, partly unconscious since they were nothing but chapters added without his knowledge to his *Monadologie*. Let us follow him in some of these stages. The conception of the infinitesimal calculus which

[1] Cf. Goblot (Ed.), *Le système des sciences*, pp. 45–6.

gradually grew up in his mind was not an entirely personal production. Without being conscious of it—at least we have no proof to the contrary—he benefited by the discoveries of his predecessors and of scientists who were almost his contemporaries. He was seeking the continuous, the indivisible. Now about 1635, the Italian Jesuit Cavalieri had the idea of measuring surfaces or volumes by cutting them by lines or planes parallel to one another, and taking the sum of the sections thus obtained ; each section is regarded as indivisible and the displacement of the cutting plane is called " flux ".[1] He would need the integral calculus ; but Pascal, whom he often quotes, had already considered a small " cut " formed by starting from a curvilinear triangle and erecting upon it a series of infinitely small prisms. Pascal, however, had not the method for arriving at the general result. Before him, Fermat had studied maxima and minima in 1629, considered the variable A of a function F, without increase, the same variable with the increase E, developed the two terms of the equation according to the powers of E, and cancelled the terms in which E appears as a factor. Hence the solution :—

$$\frac{F\ (A\ +E) - F\ (A)}{E} = 0.$$

or according to the actual notation :

$$\frac{d\ F\ (x)}{d\ x} = \mathrm{F}^1(x) = 0.$$

The differential calculus was discovered. The integral calculus was also discovered. For Fermat cut an area to be measured into segments forming a geometrical progression of which the sum is known, one term of which he causes to vanish at the end. Thus, thanks to Fermat, the differential calculus has been discovered ; thanks to Fermat and Pascal the integral calculus was glimpsed.

[1] Baron Carra de Vaux, *Leibniz*, in the series *Philosophes et Penseurs*, Paris, 1900, p. 5.

But neither one nor the other was able to generalize. It fell to Leibniz to invent the language and the symbols, and to generalize the methods sketched out by his predecessors.

On the 29th October, 1675, taking up Cavalieri's summation of indivisibles, he invented the symbol of integration, $\int$. A few days afterwards he conceived the symbol of differentiation, dx, for on the 11th November, 1675, he writes, as we do to-day, $\int y \, dy = \frac{y^2}{2}$.[1]

In December, 1675, he obtained by integration the curve of which the subnormal is equal to the ordinate ; on the 24th October, 1676, he communicated to Newton his solution of the problem of tangents by differential calculus, generalizing a rule already attained by Sluse. For that purpose he had discovered the derivatives of y^2 and y^3, etc.

$$d(y^2) = (y + dy)^2 - y^2$$
$$\text{or} \quad y^2 + 2y.dy + dy^2 - y^2 \, dy^3 = 3y^2 dy.$$

He then invented the terms differential equation and derived function. In 1683 he put forward a new method for finding maxima and minima, distinguishing the conditions by the signs $+$ and $-$. He was led to seek for " the difference of the difference ", which we now call the second differential. He generalized the formula previously found for a power of the variable $dx^a = ax^{a-1}$, by applying this formula to the negative or fractional exponent. He calls his method *Algorithme du calcul différential*. He calls the constant term appearing in an equation " the parameter ". In 1686 he studied the " Osculatory Circle " ; in 1689 he treats of the problem of the Isochrone. In 1692 he invented the terms and the notions of curvilinear co-ordinates and of envelope curves. Finally, he is the first to employ the term *function*. These results were made known to the

[1] For the integral sign see Leibniz, *Geometria recondita*, 1686.

public in a work by the Marquis de L'Hospital called *The Analysis of the Infinitely Small*, which appeared in 1696.[1]

Leibniz himself wrote between 1714 and 1716 the history of his discovery under the title *Historia et origo calculi differentialis*.

But there appeared at Paris in 1760, summing up an invention made fifty years before, a work entitled *The Method of Fluxions*, by Isaac Newton.[2] The illustrious mathematician had reached, at about the same time as Leibniz, the same conclusion by a different route. He explains the origin of his discovery as follows :

" There is close agreement between the literal operations of algebra and the numerical operations of arithmetic. Thus there is a correspondence between the decimal arithmetical fractions and algebraical terms continued to infinity. The figures placed on the right continue to diminish on a decimal scale ; the same is the case for terms arranged in uniform progression continued to infinity, according to the order of any numerator or denominator.

Decimal fractions transform vulgar fractions into whole numbers ; thus infinite series change the classes of complicated terms into simple unities. Hence I shall show how two compound quantities can be reduced to simple terms.

After this declaration of principles, Newton performs this reduction by division and by the abstraction of roots. Then he passes from the numerical equation, taken as the the first example, to an algebraic equation. He arrives at the notion of " fluent quantities ", which are considered as being augmented gradually and indefinitely.

He then establishes the relations of their fluxions, and their application to curves, obtaining the same result as Leibniz, but with a less clear terminology. The differential calculus is completed by the integral calculus ;

---

[1] Carba de Vaux, op. cit., pp. 9 and 10.
[2] Newton, *The Method of Fluxions*, London, 1736.

after the introduction of infinitely small quantities, the elimination of them, the infinitesimal calculus was brought into being.

Critical study has shown that the invention was independent on the two sides and practically simultaneous. It is not necessary for us to insist upon this point of historical order. But as regards the subject we are dealing with we may note the following points :—

(1) The method and point of departure differed in the two authors. Thus, in the first place, their independence was justified. On the other hand, once the principle had been stated, each development took place in the full light of logic. In this respect their work was conscious.

(2) But notice the circumstances which prepared their invention : On the 24th October, 1676, Newton wrote to Leibniz ; in his reply, the latter describes his solution of the problem of tangents by differential calculus ; thus the two scientists were both informed about each other's personal investigations. Thus, while proceeding with the analysis by different routes, they were able without being conscious of it to benefit, each to the profit of his methods, by an idea suggested by the other.

(3) As far as Leibniz is concerned, we may recollect that he knew of Cavalieri's " Indivisibles ", Pascal's " cut ", Fermat's quadratures and rectifications of curves. Now the principles of the differential calculus are found in the writings of Fermat, and those of the integral calculus in Pascal's. Leibniz generalized the particular solutions of his forerunners. Further, he created the language of the infinitesimal calculus, which act is again a form of generalization. That was his real invention. But in every mental operation involving generalization, there is a bringing together of objects, followed by a comparative abstraction utilizing the common elements of these objects in view of the general idea which is to result. Now this mental work is, generally speaking, unconscious. Thus what was unconscious to some extent in Leibniz's case, was the use made of the

particular solutions given by Cavalieri, Pascal, Fermat, etc., in the work of generalization from which the theory of the infinitesimal calculus arose. What was not unconscious was the logical development of the principles, once they had been formulated by the author.

5. *Monge and Descriptive Geometry*

In the case of the invention of descriptive geometry by Monge, we find again the unconscious operation of the imagination. We know that this great mind prepared the production of this fertile idea by stubborn labour. In accordance with the recommendation of Hartmann, the unconscious was awakened from its lethargy by the demand of conscious logic. The fact is so startling that at first blush, one might believe that it is a matter of entirely conscious work.

We know the initial conditions of the problem : A piece of paper has only two dimensions, length and breadth, but a real object seen in space has another in addition, height or depth. How are we to represent the three dimensions simultaneously and be able to reconstitute in an exact manner the shapes of bodies as they appear in space ? Monge considers, one after another, the point, the straight line, the plane, and projections on a plane. He imagines a single point, then its relationships to other points, A, B, C, D. He remarks that in the case of a sphere, all points have the same property with reference to the centre. But the centre is also a point. Hence, the general conclusion is reached : The position of one point is related to that of the others.

If we then pass from the point to the straight line, we remark similar properties, for the line is a series of points. In the same way a plane is a series of lines having identical properties. Now a sheet of paper is a plane. On the other hand every body is composed of points, of lines, and of planes. In order to represent a body on the paper it is therefore necessary to establish a relationship between the points on the paper and the points which make up the body : Monge conceived this relation when he devised the theory of projection.

The projection of a point on a plane will be the foot of the perpendicular to the plane drawn through that point. From this the inventor of descriptive geometry proceeds to the projection of straight lines, of surfaces, and of solid bodies.

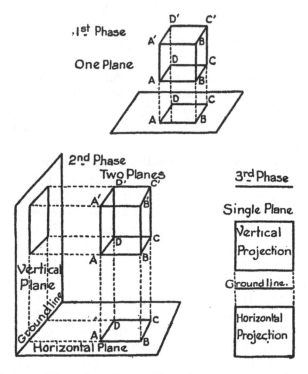

But at this point the problem becomes more difficult. The projection of a cube on a horizontal plane gives a square, that is to say, the same figure as one face of the cube. How are we to represent the cube with all its faces ? Length and breadth are shown on the horizontal plane ; we require a second plane, the vertical plane to represent height. Monge thus imagines the two planes of projection separated by the ground line.

Now these two planes may be made into one. If we turn the vertical plane around the line of intersection, the ground line, as a hinge, to bring it into the position of a continuation of the horizontal plane, we get a single plane.

We may thus distinguish three phases in this representation of solid bodies : first one plane, secondly two distinct planes, finally the two planes converted into a single one in the final working drawing, by pressing down one of the planes to a position adjacent to the other.

The principles of the new science were thus founded, and we may investigate the conscious or unconscious nature of the work thus performed. First of all, the chain of propositions, the passage from the point to the line, from the line to the plane, from surfaces to solid figures, and the successive necessity of a projection on a plane, then two projections on two planes joined together, are logical operations which were discussed at length, and hence examined in the full light of consciousness.

But these arguments were suggested one after another by dissociations and associations which prepared the formation of the mental pictures, and were for the most part unconscious ; the single plane is inconceivable without the two preceding planes ; in order to pass from the two planes to the final working drawing, it was necessary to make a clear and conscious picture of the successive moments of the pressing down. Some of these moments are represented in the following figures showing the projection of the point A.

If we turn the vertical plane towards the left the horizontal plane remaining fixed, we pass progressively to Figures 1, 2, 3, and finally to Figure 4, which represents the final working drawing ; we thus witness the disappearance of the two planes and the birth of the single plane which replaces them. It is plain that Monge did not stop at each of these stages ; in his case the final plan was elaborated as suddenly as are all images formed by the imagination. Without his having told us anything concerning the mysterious working of his mind in producing the invention, we may assert that, in a new science, built up of images, and making use of images to produce a series of deductions the part of the unconscious must have been considerable. On the one hand the unconscious imagination was responsible for the formation of the images ; on the other hand the unconscious reason produced the logical fusion of the elements of this, as of all other, mental syntheses. While at its simplest expression at the commencement of inventive construction, this latent work of the reason became greater and greater in proportion as the elements and known properties of geometrical figures became more numerous.[1]

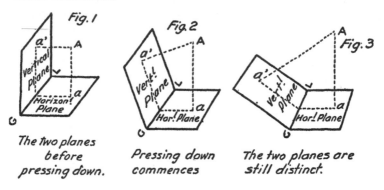

Fig. 1
The two planes before pressing down.

Fig. 2
Pressing down commences

Fig. 3
The two planes are still distinct.

6. The Statements and Examples of Laplace

Concerning the vast field formed by the application of mathematics to astronomy, we may take the evidence of Laplace, speaking as a theorist in his *Essay on Probability* and as an experimenter in his *Description of the System of the Universe.*

As a theorist he recognizes first of all that the work of the unconscious is prepared by conscious attention : " Attention to a particular quality of objects ends by endowing our organ with an exquisite sensitiveness,

[1] Monge, *Géometrie descriptive*, Paris, 1811, pp. 1 and 12.

which enables this quality to be recognized even when it becomes indistinguishable to the common run of mankind." [1]

He also recognizes the existence of the unconscious in *memory* : " The impressions which accompany memory traces serve to recall to us the cause of them. Thus in recollecting something we have been told, there is a recollection of the confidence which we place in the teller, and if his name escapes us, we find it again by recalling successively the names of those to whom we had spoken until we arrive at the name of the person who inspired us with confidence ; this proves the part played by feeling in memory. [2] He then indicates the conditions

Fig. 4

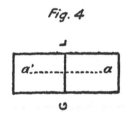

The Single Final Plane

under which this work of memory is accomplished : " Memory traces grow in intensity as a result of time and unbeknown to us. The things which we learn in the evening are engraved in the sensorium during sleep, and are easily retained by this means. I have often observed that, by ceasing to think for some days of some very complicated question, it became quite easy to me when I came to consider it afresh." This is a confession that he made progress in his power of comprehension ; but this progress is not conscious.

What is the method to be ? " Induction, analogy,

---

[1] Laplace, *Essai philosophique sur les probabilités*, Paris, 1840, p. 238.
[2] Op. cit., p. 231.

hypotheses founded on the fact and corrected by fresh observation, a happy kind of tact given us by Nature and strengthened by comparison of its indications with experience, these are the principal means of arriving at the truth." [1]

He notes the relation between habit, and the unconscious mechanism : " The operations of the *sensorium*, and the movements which it causes to be made, become easier and, as it were natural, by frequent repetition. This psychological principle explains our habits . . . The *sensorium* can receive impressions too weak to be felt, but sufficient to determine action, of the cause of which we are ignorant."

Andoyer, in his study of Laplace's scientific work, tells us how the latter faithfully applied these psychological principles to put himself into the best mental attitude for discovering and inventing : " I have always," said Laplace, " cultivated mathematics rather by reason of the taste for it than of any desire for a vain reputation, which does not interest me. My greatest amusement is to study the path of inventors, to see their genius at grips with the obstacles they meet. I then put myself in their place." [2]

This excellent state of mind is corroborated by Laplace's methods of work. " He unites powerful imagination with logical severity, and draws conclusions from unexpected relationships . . . In the universe he sees absolute determinism ; the actual state depends upon the preceding state, and is the cause of the following state." For it is a plan of the whole that he is trying to construct. That is why this scientist " had wonderful intuitions which hardly ever led him astray ; he generalized as much as possible ". In order to make no mistake in this line of work and to increase the probabilities of theory, " he lessens the number of hypotheses upon which it is founded, and increases as far as possible the number

---

[1] Op. cit., p. 247.
[2] Andoyer, *L'œuvre scientifique de Laplace*, p. 20.

of the phenomena which it explains." He proceeds by progressive extension, by increasing generalization. But he does not reach this at the first attempt. He repeatedly returns to the same subject to perfect and complete his previous work. Nor does he succeed entirely alone : he makes use of the collaboration of others, and of all researches which preceded his own, in particular those of Legendre and Lagrange. Finally, in order not to be deceived by his own hypotheses, he remarks that " a thousand chance causes can alter the march of nature : we have to consider a large number of cases in order that the effects of chance causes may cancel one another out ; the average results show us only regular and constant phenomena ".[1]

We may note this plenitude of observations with a view to invention or discovery ; we shall find it again in the case of almost all scientists ; most frequently, in fact, a new idea springs from the complicated tangle of a crowd of apparently diverse notions. In this apparition of the idea not prepared by any antecedent, there is a refined form of unconscious logic. Laplace is aware of the whole advantage to be derived from analogy.

In his *Exposition of the System of the Universe* [2] he tells us the considerations which led him to conceive his famous hypothesis of the formation of stars, planets, and satellites :—

" Although the elements of the system of planets are arbitrary, there is nevertheless between them a set of relationships which may enlighten us as to their origin. When we consider these with attention we are astonished to see that all planets move around the sun from west to east, and almost always in the same plane, satellites move round their planets in the same sense and almost in the same plane as the planets ; the sun finally, the planets and their satellites, as far as their rotational movement has been observed, turn on their own axes

[1] Op. cit., p. 92
[2] Laplace, *Exposition du systeme du monde*, Paris, an VII.

in the same sense and almost in the same plane as their orbits . . . Another equally remarkable phenomenon of the solar system is the almost circular shape of the planetary orbits, while those of comets are very much elongated. We are here compelled to recognize the effect of a regular cause . . ." [1]

To these four remarks Laplace adds two statements : " The telescope shows us nebulæ having more or less brilliant nuclei, surrounded by a nebulosity which, in condensing on the surface of the nuclei, transforms them into stars ; on the other hand the planet Saturn is surrounded by a ring which seems to indicate both its past and its future."

The astronomer asks these two questions : (1) Was not the sun originally a nebula ? (2) Are not the rings around Saturn the material for future satellites, and may not each planet have produced its satellites by means of similar rings ?

He supports his hypothesis by taking the laws of mechanics into account. In the beginning, we have a nebula endowed with rotational movement ; it cools and shrinks in volume ; this causes an increase in its speed of rotation ; this increase in speed results in rings of gaseous matter being left behind by the nebula as it contracts, in the plane of its equator. What happens around the nebula happens around the sun. The ring breaks up as it cools ; hence the planets revolving around the sun. The same phenomenon takes place in the case of the planets, resulting in satellites revolving around them. [2]

Laplace tells us that he found the first germ of this idea in Buffon. This distinguished naturalist thought that " a comet falling on the sun drove out of it a torrent of matter, hence the formation of planets and of satellites ". This explanation was obviously insufficient for a mathe-

---

[1] Op. cit., pp. 343, 344.
[2] Cf. Poincaré (H.), *Leçons sur les hypothèses cosmogoniques*, Paris, 1913, pp. 6–64.

matician such as Laplace, but it suggested research : the first unconscious action.

Need we also consider the influence of Kant ? The German philosopher had, as a matter of fact, set forth his views on the origin of the universe in a work published in 1755 under the title of *General History of Nature and Theory of the Heavens*. Now the work of Laplace appeared for the first time in 1796. It is possible that a dependence existed ; but in no place does Laplace refer to Kant. Whereas he had no hesitation in citing Buffon as follows : " Buffon is the only one known to me who since the discovery of the true system of the universe, has tried to find the way back to the origin of planets and satellites."

The ideas governing the elaboration of the cosmogony of Laplace amount to six : (1) The insufficiency of the explanations given by Buffon ; (2) The like sense of the movements of the planets ; (3) The like sense of the movements of the planets ·and their satellites ; (4) The smallness of the eccentricity of the orbits of the planets and satellites ; (5) The large eccentricity of the orbits of comets ; (6) The existence of the rings of Saturn.

The rejection of Buffon's theory excited his curiosity and stimulated research ; the five other ideas suggested analogies based on true likenesses. No one of these, taken alone, could have justified the generalization made by Laplace ; grouped together, they inspired his cosmogony. As the author tells us, the whole was not thought out on a single day. The work was done unconsciously, little by little, by reflection followed by frequent pauses. Thus,. the whole hidden part played by the unconscious when an analogy evokes the idea of a general hypothesis, is realized here ; the application of the unconscious implied by the synthetic fusion of varied elements, co-ordinated in view of a doctrine, is found to be present. What was conscious, was the considered examination of each of the five facts of which we have spoken, and the series of calculations in mechanics to which the author devoted himself ; what was unconscious, was solely the conception of the analogies, and their fusion into a definite hypothesis.

7. The Cases of Ampère and Gauss

Like Laplace, Ampère, of whom we shall have to speak at greater length when dealing with physics, recognized the influence of the unconscious in his mathematical discoveries. M. Louis de Launay, in his work Le grand Ampère, gives us this characteristic example. On the 27th April, 1802, at Bourg-en-Bresse, he gave a shout of joy. This was the reason : " It was seven years ago, says Ampère, I proposed to myself a problem which I had not been able to solve directly, but for which I had found by chance a solution, and knew that it was correct, without being able to prove it. The matter often recurred to my mind, and I had sought twenty times unsuccessfully for this solution. For some days I had carried the idea about with me continually. At last, I do not know how, I found it, together with a large number of curious and new considerations concerning the theory of probability. As I think there are very few mathematicians in France who could solve this problem in less time, I have no doubt that its publication in a pamphlet of twenty pages is a good method for obtaining a chair of mathematics in a college." [1]

In actual fact, this memoir entitled " Considerations of the mathematical theory of games of chance ", corrected in accordance with some hints from Laplace, and then twice revised by its author, brought Ampère to the Lycée at Lyons, then to the École Polytechnique, and to the Institute. We note that the prime motive of his composition was not fame, but material necessity ; Madame Julie Ampère, who lived in financial straits at Lyons, while her husband taught at Bourg, pressed him to solve and publish his problem in order to get some money from the sale of this memoir.

[1] Launay (Louis de), Le grand Ampère, Paris, 1925.

Thus the origin of this work is found in a *desire*, and even a *need*, both phenomena of feeling. The solution is felt to be correct, but the demonstration is not to be found ; intuition precedes reason ; the author seeks twenty times for the full solution ; the idea follows him about everywhere, and the discovery is thus prepared for consciously. At last the proof appeared, without his knowing how, on the 27th April, 1802, together with a whole crop of mathematical developments in the theory of probabilities : a fine piece of work performed by the unconscious thus succeeds in reaching the light. It had aimed at the essentials of the proof, for the verification of the result had already been made. fully consciously. We could repeat the same observation concerning Gauss when seeking vainly to prove a theorem in higher arithmetic for four years : " At last," he writes, " two days ago I succeeded, not by dint of painful effort, but so to speak by the grace of God. As a sudden flash of light, the enigma was solved. For my part, I am not in a position to point to the thread which joins what I knew previously and to what I have succeeded in doing." [1]

A piece of work in geometry was done by Sully Prudhomme under the same conditions. It is always prolonged unconscious work which precedes the unexpected appearance of the fertile idea.

8. *Calculators such as Inaudi have made use of Unconscious Work*

This mysterious agent also assists those conjurers of genius who play with arithmetical operations as others do with thimbles. Take the case of Inaudi. When he appeared at 24 years of age at the Academy of Sciences, he astonished everyone by the certainty and rapidity of his replies : he was found by Charcot and Binet to be an auditive type. No calculating ancestor is known in his family. Shortly before his birth, his mother had a

---

[1] Gauss, letter of 3rd September, 1805, quoted in the *Revue des questions scientifiques*, Brussels, Oct., 1884, p. 575.

mania for calculating economies to be made in order to avoid the seizure of her goods which the law threatened. This fact, reported by Inaudi's foster brother, has been cited as showing the influence of heredity, but this example of the hereditary unconscious is only pure conjecture.

Without having had any teaching, Inaudi possessed a very good head; he was, as Binet tells us, very intelligent.

Inaudi proceeded as follows. Figures were dictated, Inaudi repeated them one by one and then as a whole. He then calculated while moving about and even while replying to questions put to him. He remembered as many as three hundred figures at a sitting. If we admit, following Gall and Taine, the theory of partial memories, we have in Inaudi's case one prodigious in respect of figures. The clearness of his auditive impressions makes the work easy; he was a type at once auditive and motor. His procedure was logical. In doing a multiplication he began at the left, breaking up the operation in several steps, then suddenly the regularity of deduction gave place to intuition; he groped his way as if seeking for a word in the dictionary. The part of the unconscious in this mental calculation is said by Binet and Scripture to be as follows:—

(1) What has been retained is thought of without being articulated, in a semi-conscious manner.

(2) The multiplication of two numbers is effected before they enter into the full consciousness of our mind; there is a kind of semi-consciousness similar to that which unites the word to the sound and to the idea.

(3) Finally, through his unconscious, the calculator has an impression of the limits between which the figures sought for are comprised.[1]

Logically speaking, these simplifications are enthymemes, and psychologically the effects of habit. But,

[1] Binet, *Psychologie des grande calculateurs et des joueurs d'échecs*, pp. 101, 102.

as we have seen, the propositions assumed by the enthymeme are only partially unconscious ; on the other hand, habit reduces, but does not absolutely abolish consciousness. It is in this very relative sense that we retain the influence of the unconscious in the case of rapid calculators.

9. *The Unconscious in the case of Henri Poincaré*

These are only the lower exercises of mathematical work. In the case of the great architects of mathematical genius, such as Henri Poincaré, the mysterious work of the mind is interesting in quite another way.

Nothing could be more significant, in this respect, than the statements of the great scientist. He has given us his ideas both in *Science and Method* and in the *Matin* under the title " How Science is produced and how we invent ".[1]

Let us first consider the character of the man and see whether we cannot find traces in him of the unconscious influence of heredity. His grandfather was an apothecary, his father a doctor, his mother had a gift of order and organization ; his two great uncles were geometers. As a child, young Henri searched the sky for new stars ; his memory, like that of Inaudi, was auditive rather than visual. In his fourth year, he was already a mathematician, he distinguished himself at school by his taste for geometry. But he already showed a practical bent : he invented for amusement, he played at railways and at stage-coaches. His great principle was already that of studying nature, because we love it, and loving it because it is beautiful.[2]

When he discovered fuchsian functions, he was Professor at Caen. These functions have properties

---

[1] Poincaré, *Science et méthode*, Paris, 1908. *Le Matin*, Paris, 25th Nov., and 24th Dec., 1908.

[2] Poincaré, *Biographie analytique des écrits*. Gauthiers-Villars, 25th May, 1912.

analogous to those of elliptical functions. The number of zeros and of infinites contained in the interior of a fundamental polygon are always the same for each function. Two fuchsian functions of the same group are always united by an algebraic equation, the nature of which coincides with the geometrical nature of the group ; hence we have a point of contact with algebraic functions. From this results the following important theorem : the co-ordinates at the points of an algebraic curve defined in any manner whatever can always be expressed by uniform functions of a parameter ; they are thus an instrument for the theory of abelian integrals.

These mathematical details are sufficient to show that these functions, linked as they are both to algebra and geometry, are the result of various combinations. Poincaré was able to connect them with arithmetic itself. That is to say that his discovery, produced by bringing together the results of several sciences, is a *true invention.*

This being so, we may follow the author himself in the account which he gives of his researches.

" For a fortnight, I had been trying to prove that no function could exist analogous to what I have since called the fuchsian function. I was very ignorant at that time ; every day I sat down at my table ; I passed an hour or two there : I tried a great number of combinations, but I did not reach any result. One evening, I drank some black coffee, which I was not accustomed to do ; I could not sleep ; ideas crowded in on me ; they seemed to me to collide with one another, until two of them hooked together, as it were, to form a stable combination. In the morning I had established the existence of one class of fuchsian functions, that derived from the hyper-geometric series ; I had nothing to do but to check the result, which took me a few hours . . .

" At this time I left Caen where I was living at the time, to take part in a course of Geology. The journey made me forget my mathematical work ; when we arrived at Coutances we got into an omnibus to make some excursion or other ; at the moment of putting my foot on the step, the idea occurred to me, without anything in my immediately preceding thoughts having prepared me for it, that the transformations which I have used to define fuchsian functions were identical with those of non-euclidian geometry. I did not verify this : I had no time to do so, since no sooner was I seated in the omnibus than I took up the conversation I had begun ; but I was entirely certain of the result. On returning to Caen I verified it at leisure, in order to satisfy my conscience.

" I then set to work to study arithmetical questions without any apparent result of importance, and without suspecting that there would be the least connection with my previous researches. Disgusted with my failure, I went for a few days' holiday to the seaside and thought of quite other matters. One day, while walking on the cliffs, the idea occurred to me, *again with the same characteristics of brevity, suddenness and certitude* (I underline these words) that arithmetical transformations of indefinite ternary quadritic form were identical with those of non-euclidian geometry, Here was a new problem. At first all my efforts only served to teach me the difficulty more fully. This part of the work was entirely *conscious*. It was again followed by unconscious work . . .

" This was followed by my departure for Mont-Valérien where I had to perform my military service ; I thus had very different preoccupations. One day, whilst crossing the street, the solution of the difficulty which had stopped me appeared to me quite suddenly. I did not attempt to go into it more deeply at once, and it was only after my service that I took the question up again. I was in possession of all the elements, and only needed to assemble and arrange them."

After this very circumstantial account Poincaré adds, in order to characterize these facts of the unconscious :—

" What will strike you at first are these appearances
of sudden illumination which are the manifest tokens of
a long unconscious labour which has preceded them ;
the part played by this unconscious labour in mathematical invention appears incontestible to me, and
traces will be found of it in other cases where it is less
evident.   Often, when one is working at a difficult
question, one produces nothing of any use on the first
occasion of attacking the problem ; later, one may
take a rest of greater or less duration, and sit down
at the table again.   For the first half hour one may
continue to get no result, and then quite suddenly
the decisive idea is presented to the mind.   One could
say that conscious labour had been more fruitful because
it has been interrupted and because the rest had restored
to the mind its power and freshness.   It is more probable
that the period of rest is filled by unconscious labour,
and that the result of this labour is afterwards revealed
quite suddenly to the geometer, as in the cases that
I have cited ; only that the revelation, instead of
appearing during a walk or a journey, has been produced
during a period of conscious work, but independently
of this work, which plays at the most the part of a
releasing force, acting as a stimulus which excites the
results already attained during the rest period, but still
buried in the unconscious, to take a conscious form."

Finally, we may cite his opinion concerning the cause
which decides the appearance of one invention rather
than another :—

" The demonstration which takes form is that which
has most affinity to our æsthetic feeling.   Only those
combinations which move us attract our attention :
The unconscious is what brings about affinity between
our feeling and invention ; useful combinations are
precisely those which are most beautiful.[1]

" Why should this importance be attached to beauty ?

---

[1] Poincaré (H.), *Science et méthode*, pp. 56–8.

It is because beauty is the expression of order. Now a mathematical demonstration is a series of syllogisms placed in a certain order. The order is more important than the syllogisms themselves. The intuition or feeling for order is necessary for inventing them. Mathematical invention does not consist in making new combinations of mathematical entities already known, it does not consist in constructing useless combinations, but in constructing those which are useful, and which form only a minute minority. That is why in view of the multitude of facts which are presented to us it is necessary to retain only those *giving a large yield, privileged phenomena* which have more effect on our feeling. This sensibility of ours acts as a sieve. During the period of apparent rest and unconscious labour, these future elements of our combination, like the hooked atoms of Epicurus, are set in motion. Preliminary conscious labour has mobilized some of these atoms. During unconscious labour, these atoms continue their dance and enter into combination among themselves or with other atoms. Those combinations which have a chance of succeeding are those where one element is one of the atoms freely chosen by our will." [1]

From these statements of H. Poincaré, and from the account given of his life by Frédéric Masson, at his reception at the Academie Française on the 28th January, 1909, we may set down the following points :—

(1) The hereditary unconscious predisposed him to scientific invention ; his grandfather an apothecary, his father a doctor, his mother fond of order, his two great uncles geometers, his various forefathers are evidently persons in love with scientific precision.

(2) In his case, conscious labour only took place when prepared by a long conscious incubation. In fact, for more than a fortnight, he passed an hour or two every day in making combinations without getting any results.

(3) Unconscious inspiration was thus preceded by some days of conscious work—first at Caen, then at the

[1] Ibid.

seaside, finally at Mont-Valérien. The solution sought for followed upon entirely conscious preliminary work.

(4) The discovery or invention springs up from the depths of the unconscious like an inspiration, always having the same characteristic of brevity, suddenness, and certitude. At Caen, on the cliffs, and also at Mont-Valérien there was actual discontinuity between the preceding conscious work and the flash of inspiration.

(5) Fresh conscious labour is necessary for verifying the discovery and developing its consequences. At Caen, the discovery of the fuchsian function was made in the morning, and verification took place on the following day. At Mont Valérien the inspiration came in the street, and it was verified much later during military service.

(6) The psychological process of invention in Poincaré's case is as follows : The conscious labour prepares for the unconscious ; it mobilizes in some way the elements presented to the unconscious. This last does not act as an automaton ; it does not furnish ready-made results, but only *inspirations, points of departure*. Calculations are performed consciously. Finally, the rôle of the unconscious is not that of furnishing a rational process excluding less rational combinations, nor a process of calculation solving the problem in all its details : It is solely an inspiration issuing from the realm of feeling.[1]

10. *A Small Personal Experience*

Professors of mathematics are unanimous in saying that they make from time to time fortunate hits which are not matters of genius, but are unforeseen. I have had this experience myself. I have already found several times, on waking in the morning, solutions or explanations which I had vainly sought for on the preceding evening. Here is how, one fine morning, I caught sight of a new demonstration of a well-known

[1] Cf. Dwelshauvers, op. cit., p. 54.

theorem : The sum of the three angles of a triangle is equal to two right angles. Here we are evidently dealing with a triangle in a space of three dimensions, and not with the triangle in hyper-space.

The classical demonstration is well known. The straight line *BN* (Fig. 1) parallel to *AC* determines the following pairs of equal angles :—

4 = 2 (alternate internal angles).

3 = 5 (corresponding angles).

Hence the series 1 + 4 + 5 is equal to the series 1 + 2 + 3.

But the sum 1 + 4 + 5 is equal to two right angles (adjacent angles on the same side of the straight line

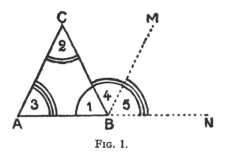

FIG. 1.

AN). Hence the sum 1 + 2 + 3, being equal to the preceding sum, is also equal to two right angles.

This reasoning is impeccable ; because it is justified by three propositions proved previously in all systems of geometry :—

(1) The adjacent angles situated on the same side of the straight line are supplementary.

(2) The alternate internal angles formed by two parallel straight lines cut by a third are equal.

(3) Corresponding angles formed under the same conditions are also equal.

These three proofs, preceding the proposition in question, satisfy our reason completely.

But like many geometrical solutions, it has a fault :

it establishes the result without making it self-evident ;
it is apodictic without being representative. It gives a
rational proof but presents nothing to the imagination.
We know that the sum of the three angles is equal to
two right angles, but we do not see the two right angles.

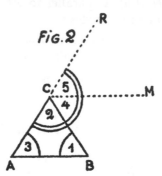

We ought therefore to construct two right angles and
show in our proof their equality to those of the triangle.
In order to get this result I tried in vain various constructions but only modified the classical demonstration.

In Fig. 2 we have

> 1 = 4 alternate internal angles.
> 3 = 5 (corresponding angles).

Whence

> 1 + 2 + 3 = 2 + 4 + 5 = two right-angles.

But we do not see the two right angles. Another proof
which does not satisfy the imagination is as follows :—

In Fig. 3, MN being parallel to AB we have

> 4 = 3 (alternate internal angles).
> 5 = 1 (alternate internal angles).

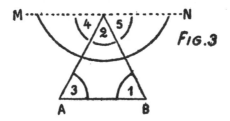

Thus the sum 4 + 2 + 5 which is equal to two right angles is equal to the sum 1 + 2 + 3 of the angles of the triangle. But we still do not see the two right angles.

But after having well thought over these various unsatisfying combinations, I gave up thinking about it and went to sleep. In the morning, without an effort, as if by chance I pictured to myself the two right angles constructed at the extremities A and B at the base of the triangle, and, thanks to the straight line CD drawn parallel to the two perpendiculars AN and BN, I saw immediately the following equalities (Fig. 4) :—

1 = 2 (alternate internal angles).

4 = 3 (alternate internal angles).

Hence 1 + 4 = 2 + 3 = C, and

5 + 6 + 1 + 4 = 5 + 6 + 2 + 3 = 5 + 6 + C

= two right angles.

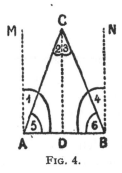

FIG. 4.

Thus the three angles of the triangle were equal to the sum of the two right angles. It was both a demonstration for the mind and a construction for the eyes. The unconscious work carried out during sleep had completed the conscious efforts of the night before. A curious fact was that the figure representing the two right angles, a figure that I had sought for so industriously on the evening before, first appeared to me quite suddenly : the very easy proof of the construction was done a minute or two after the representation of this figure. Here is a little invention—so elementary that it would make a Poincaré smile—which establishes clearly the following points :—

(1) It was preceded by a great desire and prepared for by conscious combinations.

(2) There was discontinuity between conscious labour and unconscious labour.

(3) The construction of the figure with the two right angles, was the result of the unconscious labour and was a synthetic vision, an intuition.

(4) But the proof, rapid as it was, was made subsequently to the intuition and was conscious.

Summary

We may here conclude this inquiry in the domain of the mathematical sciences. It allows us to set down the following results :—

(1) The unconscious appears in its *hereditary* form in the case of the four Cassinis, who were mathematicians from father to son [1] ; in the case of the three Bernoullis, Jacques, Jean, and Daniel (the two first were brothers, the third was the nephew of Jean) ; in the case of Euler and his children, who were all mathematicians in various degrees [2] ; perhaps in the calculator Inaudi, whose case we have examined ; finally in the case of a great many others, notably Henri Poincaré, as we have shown.

(2) This unconscious incubation is prepared for by conscious labour in different ways. In the case of Pascal, by the ardent desire for discovery ; in the case of Leibniz by the reasoned utilization of the discoveries of his predecessors ; in the case of Laplace by proof of the mistakes made by Buffon ; in the case of Ampère by the need to earn his living, in the pursuit of fame ; in the case of Poincaré, Leibniz, Pascal, and Ampère, by conscious research, but in other fields than mathematics (for example, in chemistry, in geology, in biology)

[1] Coursat, *Vie et travaux des savants modernes*, Paris, 1923, p. 49.
[2] Op. cit., p. 82.

research which furnished an indirect stimulus to the projected invention ; in every case by obstinate labour carried out consciously and for a long period, but ordered with regard to the solution sought for.

(3) There was, however, *discontinuity* between conscious preparation and unconscious incubation. Pascal passed from one research to another apparently unmethodically, apart from the case of his calculating machine ; Leibniz interrupted his study of the infinitely small by studies in law, metaphysical discussions, and theological controversies. His invention, which was begun in 1675, was finished between 1714 and 1716, at which time his *Historia et origo calculi differentialis* appeared.[1] Laplace, so he tells us, only arrived at his *System of the Universe* by reflection, in successive stages, followed by many pauses. Ampère " sought twenty times " for the full solution of his problem, then set his mind to something else, whereupon a flash of inspiration suddenly brought light ; Poincaré was distracted from the work on his researches when on the cliffs at Caen and at Mont-Valérien ; I myself, in the little experience which I have described, only saw my fourth demonstration in the morning, after a sleep preceded by conscious work.

(4) What is the nature of this unconscious labour which is accomplished in the minds of the scientists ? In the case of Descartes and Monge, it was an imaginative elaboration resulting in the formation of a mental image ; in the case of Leibniz and Laplace, it was reasoning by analogy which was sketched out and which resulted in a great generalization ; in the majority of cases, notably in that of Poincaré, the result was revealed in the form of a *sudden illumination, a quick flash, a fortuitous intuition*. It was, as it were, the crystallization of an idea, not reasoning properly so called.

(5) Conscious reasoning always resumes its rights : inspiration is followed by conscious labour. Laplace made use of the laws of mechanics to verify very fully

[1] Carra de Vaux, op. cit., p. 10.

the exactness of the hypothesis which he had built up ; Ampère verified his problem many times before publishing it ; he had even to partially correct it as a result of suggestions made by Laplace, to whom he had submitted it ; Poincaré had no difficulty in verifying the truth of his solution when once his military service had been finished. Thus the work of conscious verification is the prolongation, or fully developed analysis, of the inventive work sketched by the unconscious and flashed into consciousness as synthesized into an idea.

This is the harvest of results which we have derived from the mathematicians. In their case, the very limited field of experience in the immense field of deduction, admit the unconscious. The following chapter allows us to expect similar findings in the case of the physical sciences, in which numerous experiments prepare the ways for laws, and where laws are extended by mathematical developments.

CHAPTER III

THE UNCONSCIOUS AND INVENTION IN THE PHYSICAL SCIENCES

The place of the unconscious in these sciences—Invention by collaboration—Inventions connected with universal gravitation—With atmospheric pressure—With light— With electricity—The invention of matches—The invention of experimental phonetics—Conclusion.

1. *The Place of the Unconscious in these Sciences*

THE mathematical sciences are of necessity logical; invention in this domain has most often the character of absolutely rational combination; if the unconscious finds its way into it, it is by penetrating into the various forms of reasoning.

On the other hand, the physical sciences are sciences of nature as it exists. Consequently, they are not any more necessary than the world, the movements and transformations of which they rule. Now this world is contingent ; if it has the form which we know it to have, it might also have another one. From this it follows that its laws cannot be set forth *a priori*, independently of the fact. They are, to quote the thought of Leibniz which was taken up again by Boutroux, "subsidiary maxims established by God." This means that these laws require to be discovered, and then checked by facts ; experiment and induction are the essential methods of the physical sciences. The unconscious can intervene in experimental procedure and in the work of induction ; we shall seek its traces in elaboration of hypotheses and in the comparison of facts by analogy.

2. Invention by Collaboration

But precisely on account of the extreme importance of experiment, the result of which may be known to many people, the inventions in physical sciences have still less of a personal character than the combinations of the mathematician. The physicist or the chemist taking up one by one the attempts of his predecessors, sometimes consciously, often unconsciously, pursues the researches of a forerunner. They take a larger view of the question, they see it from a higher level, for they see it from further away. This consideration shows us that in the territory of natural sciences inventions will be made, for the great part, in collaboration.

3. Inventions relating to Universal Gravitation

We shall find the first example of this in the discovery of universal gravitation. Before Newton's time, Galilei found that the law of the fall of bodies is the same as that of the generation of squares ; it is proportional to the square of the time taken. We are dealing here with terrestrial gravitation. Huyghens then discovered that weight diminishes with the distance from the centre of the earth, or in proportion to our elevation above the surface of the earth ; we are still dealing with terrestrial attraction. Newton studied for many years the revolutions of the planets and showed that the attractive force exercised by the sun on every body in the system varies inversely as the square of the distance ; but this phenomenon remained isolated in his mind. Thus Galilei and Huyghens had studied consciously the law of terrestrial attraction ; Newton, also consciously, had grasped the relation which expresses the attraction of celestial bodies ; he had only the most superficial notions concerning terrestrial weight. The above data constituted the conscious preparation for his discovery.

One day at his country house of Woolsthorpe, while

seated under an apple-tree, he saw an apple fall in front of him. Suddenly an analogy crossed his mind : " Why," he said to himself, " should not this power act on the moon and attract it towards the earth ? " [1] This was the flash of identification. He knew that the sun attracted the planets. He had just discovered that the attraction which binds the sun to the planets is identical with that which binds bodies to the centre of the earth. Thus, what took place unconsciously was the sudden identification of the two phenomena established in the mind of the scientist. It had that character of suddenness already noted in the case of H. Poincaré when inventing fuchsian functions. As logical continuity requires, a latent work had been done, resulting in the flash of identification between the apperception of the first law—celestial attraction—and the apperception which had for its object the identification of terrestrial attraction, and the attraction of the heavenly bodies. But so far only an hypothesis existed. After being prepared for by conscious labour, this anticipation of the law was to be confirmed by a second process of conscious labour. Newton verified the law by calculation. He made use of the value then assumed for the act of the meridian. The result did not agree, and he made up his mind to give up his great idea. But in 1682 the Academy of Sciences in Paris obtained, four years afterwards, a more correct value for the meridian.[2] This time, the verification as re-calculated by Newton, using the new value for the meridian, was a complete success. It was confirmed by an experiment made by von Jolly, Professor at Munich, about 1880.

As we see, the verification of the hypotheses, a long

[1] Cf. Sortais, *Études de philosophie sociale*, pp. 319. The accuracy of this anecdote of the apple has been doubted. But Pemberton, who was a contemporary and friend of Newton, reported it and had no reason for inventing it.

[2] This new measurement was made by Picard in the name of the Academy of Sciences. Cf. Joly, *Psychologie des grands hommes*, pp. 190–3.

and difficult process, often interrupted, was completely *conscious*. The totality of this theory of universal attraction, prepared by Galilei and by Huyghens, elaborated by Newton, and completely verified by Newton and by von Jolly, is more than a discovery; as a combination of two physical theories concerning attraction, and a comparison and identification of these theories, it is a true invention.

4. Inventions based upon Atmospheric Pressure

The solidarity of inventions is still more manifest if we study those derived from that great discovery in physics, the pressure of the atmosphere. Here also, we observe the alternation between conscious preparation, unconscious elaboration, and conscious verification.

Since the earliest antiquity the fact has been known that water rises in syringes, pumps, etc. The explanation given was that *nature abhorred a vacuum*. Aristotle and Roger Bacon deny the existence of an absolute vacuum; Galilei, noting that pumps cannot raise water to a greater height than 32 or 33 feet, concludes that "nature abhors a vacuum, but only up to a certain point". In one direction or another, we find a tendency to eliminate this illusory cause—the vacuum. There was thus at the origin of these researches a *lively desire*.

In 1643 Torricelli did his famous experiment with his barometric tube. The mercury rose to a height of 76 centimetres; now the tube had an area of 1 sq. centimetre; the weight of mercury raised was therefore $76 \times 1 \times 13 \cdot 6 = 1033 \cdot 6$ grammes. But Galilei had already proved that air has weight. This mercury therefore must represent the weight of the air resting upon 1 sq. centimetre, since there is a vacuum in the upper part of the tube. It is thus the weight of the atmosphere which causes the mercury to rise : the theory of nature's horror of a vacuum is thus disposed of.

Everything about this experiment of Torricelli appears

to be conscious. He reasons concerning its result in such a manner that the conclusion appears like that of a proved theorem.

Why, however, did he make this experiment? Why did he use the tube? Why did he use mercury, the density of which is well known? Because he had a presentiment of the result. Torricelli verified consciously an hypothesis which was elaborated more or less unconsciously in his mind. This apparatus is already a miniature barometer, and the form of this barometer appeared suddenly to the mind of the scientist as being necessary to verify a law which was not yet formulated. This is where we find clear traces of the unconscious.

This verification, made by using mercury, is not general. If the law is accurate, then, seeing that liquids have different densities and that the atmospheric pressure is sensibly constant at a given moment, the height to which the barometric liquid will rise will be the greater, the lighter the liquid. When tried with water, and then with wine, Torricelli's experiment was completely successful. In faithful adherence to Bacon's method, he multiplied and varied the conditions of the experiment. He repeated his attempts at Paris, at Rouen, and at the Puy de Dome, with his brother-in-law Périer. He came to two conclusions : (1) The cause of the rise of any liquid is the atmospheric pressure. (2) This pressure diminishes as we go up in the air. The theory of atmospheric pressure thus became general. It led to the invention of the barometer, which serves two useful purposes : (1) It indicates changes of pressure. (2) It tells us, with a sufficient degree of accuracy, at what height we are above sea-level.

We see that if Torricelli experimented with a certain degree of unconsciousness as to the result, Pascal, who prolonged and generalized his predecessor's experiments, confirmed the results consciously. Thus the study of atmospheric pressure comprises elaboration which was partly conscious and partly unconscious, and fully conscious verification, both in the case of Torricelli as of Pascal. All barometers which are modifications of Torricelli's tube are so many inventions derived from the fundamental theory of atmospheric pressure. They are new verifications, which are conscious or unconscious according as their inventors have had their minds on the first barometer, Torricelli's tube, when constructing their apparatus. First we have Fortin's barometer with a movable cistern, the syphon barometer having a curved tube, the dial barometer having a small weight pushed by variations in the level of the mercury and moving a needle on a dial, the metallic barometer of Vidi, in which the atmospheric pressure causes a metallic membrane to bend, the movements of which are transmitted by means of a lever to a needle moving on a dial ; the recording barometer, in which metal boxes deformed by the pressure of the air communicate with a pen which traces a curve of their deformations on a moving piece of paper. In all these apparatus we find the pressure of the air made use of, either by means of mercury or by an elastic metal.

The invention of the manometer must evidently also be connected with the theory of atmospheric pressure, since the gasses and vapours exercise pressure upon mercury or upon an elastic metal. Torricelli's tube is not merely a barometer, it is also a manometer.

5. *Inventions connected with Light*

We may begin with photography. The period of conscious preparation was long ; it was occupied by the successive contributions of various seekers. In 1799 Watt tried to fix luminous images but did not succeed. In 1802 Wedgewood, Davy, and Charles obtained silhouettes of opaque bodies on paper impregnated with nitrate of silver. It was impossible at that time to obtain clear images, as the light blackened the paper uniformly. The procedure was that of photographic drawing, a first step, the insufficiency of which suggested future transformation. In 1813 lithography, invented by Senefelder, of Munich, spread to France. The chance had come; Nicephore Niepce tried to perfect the technique of it and, with his son Isidore, copied engravings. This was a long and painful labour. He attempted to save himself the trouble of drawing them. Here was a need which suggested an improvement. He sought for the action of light on protected varnishes in order to be able to copy prints automatically. For this purpose, he made use of the camera obscura, which had been known since the thirteenth century; he stopped down the aperture of the lenses in order to obtain sharper images.

At this moment, by chance, he discovered a remarkable property of asphaltum or bitumen. This substance, like bichromated gelatine, is insoluble in its solvent, spirit of turpentine, when it has been exposed to the action of the sun's rays. He therefore spread some bitumen on a steel surface and placed upon it an engraving, rendered translucent by means of a fatty substance. After exposure to light for two hours he washed the plate with essence of lavender; the bitumen dissolved excepting where it had been exposed; there was thus a white image formed on the bitumen. He made a proof on a heliographic board and obtained an exact copy of the engraving. He perfected his method, and in 1822 he had produced real photography.

In the meantime Louis Jacques Mande Daguerre, a painter and decorator, had been pursuing the same ends. He got into communication with Niepce. Up to that point he had installed at Paris an original diorama, a kind of perfected panorama in which variable lighting added mobility of effect to the sense of aerial perspective. An unforeseen observation led him to the invention of the Daguerreotype.

One day he covered a plate of silvered copper with bromide of silver; he put this plate at the bottom of a dark chamber, and then exposed it to the action of light.

H

Finally he put this plate into a cupboard, without thinking of some mercury which was also in the cupboard.

On the following day, he was surprised to observe that certain parts of the plate had been altered ; the latent image had appeared. What was the cause of this appearance of the latent image ? Daguerre, on examining the cupboard, found a vessel containing mercury there. The idea came to him immediately, *a sudden and genuine flash of inspiration*, that the vapours of mercury had caused the modification and the appearance of the image. Two further tests, repetitions of this experiment, once with mercury, and the second time without it, demonstrated that the mercury was quite truly the developer of the image.

The development of Niepce's researches was thus due to Daguerre. Mercury was replaced by oxalate of iron, by pyrogallic acid, etc., but the essential thing was discovered. Variations became numerous : in 1839 Bayard replaced the metallic plate by paper ; in 1839 to 1841 the Englishman Talbot produced his photographic designs on paper, and, in order to get a positive image, recopied his negative design on a second paper sensitized by silver iodide. In 1846 Niepce de Saint-Victor, cousin of Nicéphore Niepce, invented photography on glass. Finally in 1907, Professor Korn, making use of the properties of selenium, invented telephotography. All these transformations were conscious ; they were modifications of photography properly so called.

In the history of this invention, therefore, we have the conscious preparations and trials reaching from 1799 to 1822 ; we find traces of unconscious surprise in the discovery by Niepce of the properties of asphaltum, and in the unexpected discovery by Daguerre of the developer in the form of mercury. Finally, all applications which have been made subsequently of these fundamental discoveries have been conscious derivations from them. Briefly then, photography was begun in full consciousness with the study of the decomposition of the salts of silver by luminous rays, continued with the discovery of developers by semi-conscious work, and developed and expanded finally by fully conscious logic.[1]

From photography we may pass to cinematography. The invention of this wonderful apparatus, which gives the illusion of movement, and therefore of life, allows of the observation of unconscious logic.

The study of optics revealed the principle of it ; the impression produced by light upon the eye persists for one-tenth of a second after the disappearance of the luminous body. If the retinal images succeed one another more rapidly than that, they are blotted out ; we have not a series of luminous sensations, but instead a single sensation. This result is necessarily obtained if the impressions are repeated at intervals of time less than one-tenth of a second. In this case, the eye joins the successive impressions one to another, and we have the illusion of movement. The apparatus, which was first called the Chronophotograph, is thus also a Kineto-scope or a Cinematograph.

The invention had a predecessor. In 1899 Marcy had tried to project animated images by employing perforated bands. But success had not followed the attempt. The brothers Auguste and Louis Lumière, of Lyons, were the first to effect modern cinematography. By means of a series of inventions, improvements, and successive modifications, they revolutionized the methods and the apparatus. They created the cinema.

The theory of this apparatus was elaborated little by little. Conscious preparation existed in evoking the memory of these two facts of experience : (1) If a glowing coal is rapidly revolved, we get the impression of a luminous circle. (2) This appearance of continuity is only possible when the sensations follow one another at a less interval than a tenth of a second. Now an animated scene may

[1] Cf. Bouillet, *Dictionn. Univers. des lettres, des sciences et des arts*, 1896, p. 1265. *Dictionn. encyclop. et biograph. des arts indust.*, t. 7, p. 267.

be decomposed into a series of drawings or photographs similar to one another. If then these pictures pass before the eye with a rapidity as great as that we have mentioned, they give the impression of movement.

The unconscious phenomenon resides in this illusion of movement of the whole. If the scene was decomposed into a thousand pictures which succeeded one another slowly, the consciousness would perceive a thousand distinct impressions, but if we accelerate the passage of the images, our attention fails to detect the necessary distinction between the different movements of the representation. The series appears continuous because our attention fails, that is to say, through operation of the unconscious.

But there is more to be said. In the case of the creators of the apparatus, we can distinguish three phases in the realization of this invention : (a) A completely conscious phase ; before imagining cinematography they studied the speed of light and the interval of time necessary to make several luminous sensations distinct. (b) A semi-conscious phase : quite suddenly the following idea came to them, that if the images succeeded one another very quickly one would have a single sensation, one would have luminous continuity. This idea was like a conclusion drawn suddenly from previous conscious reasoning, a sort of enthymeme, of which we have previously studied the partially unconscious character. (c) A fully conscious further phase : the apparatus had been realized by taking into account all necessary conditions as above.

Another property of light is that of polarization. Here we are dealing with the discoveries properly so called and not with an invention. We must nevertheless allude to it, for this discovery led its author Malus, to the invention of the repeating goniometer.

This is how Biot relates to us the circumstances which brought about the discovery which was the basis of the invention. In the first place, it was preceded by profound studies which were conscious operations. Malus studied refraction. A single luminous ray penetrating obliquely into any transparent body is bent at the point at which it enters the body. He knew the law of double refraction enunciated by Fresnel, and by Huyghens as follows : " If the refracting body is neither an octahedron nor a cube, every ray of light penetrating the crystal is divided into two refracted rays, one of which, the ordinary ray, follows the ordinary law of refraction given by Descartes, and the other, the extraordinary ray, follows a much more complicated law studied by Huyghens in the case of rhomboidal calcium carbonate, or Iceland Spar ; finally, the ray which has been refracted in the ordinary or extraordinary manner by a crystal, has suffered certain changes in its properties. These changes appear if it is made to traverse a second crystal ; it then suffers sometimes ordinary refraction alone, sometimes extra-ordinary refraction alone, and sometimes partly one and partly the other, according to the sense in which the faces of the second crystal are presented to it.

" Malus, who was continually occupied with the subject of double refraction, was looking one evening in Paris through his crystal prisms at the Luxembourg Palace, from the windows of which the rays of the setting sun were strongly reflected. Turning round the prism *unthinkingly* in his fingers, as he was accustomed to do continually in these observations, he noticed that one of the two images transmitted showed variations of intensity at different phases of the movement : a thing that would certainly not have happened if he had thus looked at a direct light, that of a candle, for example . . . On the next day, when again observing the same phenomenon, he recognized that it only took place completely under a certain definite inclination of the ray relatively to the reflecting surfaces. It was thus the inclination of the ray to the surface which produced it."

Here we have the phase of surprise, which results in an hypothesis of which the scientist had not yet thought : the variations in intensity of the ray depend upon the inclination of the ray to the surface. Formulated thus the law is general : the expression of it has been suggested solely by an unconscious activity of the mind. For the experiments were still insufficient to allow a generalization to be made ; the mind anticipates, by semiconscious working, the result of trials which will be renewed.

Malus then undertook the verification absolutely consciously. Since, by hypothesis, the variations of intensity of the ray depend on the angle of inclination of the ray to the crystal, he "calculated this angle according to the position in which the sun must have been in at the time when he made his discovery, and he succeeded in producing the same phenomenon with all sorts of lights and on any kind of transparent substances. This tendency of light to experience a single refraction when it traverses in a certain way bodies which exercise double refraction on ordinary light, constitute what Malus called " the polarization of light ".[1] The angle of inclination of the ray to the crystal is very important. Malus invented the repeating goniometer in order to make this measurement convenient.

To sum up, in this case we find the unconscious, neither in the preliminary studies of refraction, nor in the many verifications carried out with various lights and various substances, nor in the invention of the apparatus for measuring angles which was an application of the previous discovery. Thus, a long period of conscious work had preceded and followed unconscious elaboration ; in this latter, the extent and duration of which should not be exaggerated, simply suggested as hypothesis the law, which then became a matter for conscious verification.

The case of Foucault is very interesting. He was a great physicist but not much of a mathematician, yet he foresaw a mathematical conclusion without being able to prove it, because it answered his lively desire to demonstrate a truth which interests both the physicist

[1] Cf. Biot, *Melanges scientifiques et littéraires*, quoted by Goursat, *La vie et les travaux des savants modernes*, pp. 250-2.

and the astronomer, and to invent the pendulum which bears his name.

Foucault set himself to demonstrate the rotation of the earth ; he did some spherical trigonomometry on a small sphere of wood, and asked questions of the geometers. One day, in the Luxembourg Gardens, he met and questioned his friend Josef Bertrand ; he begged him to calculate a very small angle which was defined with precision by a geometrical construction on the little sphere. Bertrand, by making use of the similarity of spherical triangles, found that it was proportional to the sine of the latitude. " I was certain that it was," said Foucault, and his face was lit up for an instant by a flash of triumph and joy.[1] Thereupon the illustrious physicist devoted himself to long researches, a matter of conscious work. To demonstrate the rotation of our planet would be easy if he were able to measure scientifically a very small angle : he had an intuition of its value, but he could not verify this intuition, because he did not know the proof which performed its verification. This intuition of the conclusion was thus the result of unconscious work. The collaboration of Bertrand and the application of the result to the required demonstration was done fully consciously.

6. *Inventions relating to Electricity*

Let us now take the case of the inventor of electro-dynamics. Ampère, of whom we have already spoken in connection with mathematical invention, is a striking example of the combination of conscious or subconscious influences resulting in a great invention.

In his case the period of preparation, at times conscious, at others unconscious, was long and varied. He had received some lessons from his father : as a child he had

[1] Bertrand (J.), *Eulogy of Foucault*, quoted by Loridan, op. cit., p. 77.

a passion for Buffon's *Natural History*; very soon the reading of Thomas' *Eulogy of Descartes* was a revelation to him; at the age of thirteen he read Clairvant's *Algebra*, and treatises on Conic Sections by La Chapelle and l'Hôpital. His inventive faculty was already evident, for with the elementary knowledge he had acquired he composed the *Treatise on Conic Sections.* He went further, not understanding the infinitesimal calculus from the articles in the *Encyclopædia*, he had it explained to him by Daburon. He learnt physics with Professor Mollet. But from the start, physics alone did not satisfy his passion for learning. We see him in turn a botanist, a linguist dreaming of a universal language, a mathematician, a poet composing an epic poem entitled *L'Americide*, then a chemist, in contact with Davy, and above all a metaphysician. Ampère was urged on by an imperious necessity to produce, and allowed his mind to play over the most various objects. This diversity of knowledge was to become for him a latent source of inventive combination. Being filled with enthusiasm for new theories, he explored those of Gall, of Lavater, animal magnetism, spiritism, etc. We may say that his character is that of an enthusiast who always combined sentiment with scientific research. " He does not know," said M. de Launay, " how to resist any intellectual desire, nor how to follow two ideas at a time. The new thought takes complete mastery of him like a passion for a woman and possesses him entirely for a period . . . In his powerful and tortured brain, there was a disordered invasion of all the human sciences, of chemistry, physics, mathematics, zoology, botany, geology, all mixed together with metaphysics and amorous torments." [1]

Such were the antecedent circumstances, which, in Ampère's case were to have their unconscious effect in the elaboration of electro-dynamics, and the invention of the electro-magnet.

[1] Louis de Launay, op. cit., pp. 153, 154.

The following was the event which started his inventive effort in this direction :—

On the 4th September, 1820, Arago reported to the Institute the experiment performed by Oerstedt, Professor at Copenhagen. " Oerstedt had announced to his pupils the experiment he was going to make. He took a compass needle, placed it near a voltaic pile, and waited until the magnetic needle had come to rest. Then taking the connecting wire which was traversed by the current of the pile, he placed it above the compass needle, carefully avoiding any kind of shock. The needle, as everyone saw, moved." [1] It deviated from its position of equilibrium.

Oerstedt simply observed the fact. Ampère and Arago set to work to elucidate the whole matter of electro-magnetism.

The identification of the two phenomena immediately flashed through Ampère's mind. It was known that a magnetized needle obeyed the action of the earth or a magnet. It had just been discovered that an electric current had a similar action on this needle. Ampère, at a glance, brings these two facts together : (1) A current acts like a magnet ; (2) Hence a magnet and a current can be substituted one for the other. But the current directs a magnetized needle ; hence the magnet should be able to direct a movable current ; thus magnets are currents.

All these conclusions were seen by rapid intuition, previous to practical verification by the author.

Feeling sure of the conclusion which had flashed on his mind, Ampère sought for the experimental consequences of it. He wrote to his son at Geneva :—

" All my time has been taken up by one of the most important happenings of my life. Since I heard for the first time news of the beautiful discovery made by M. Oerstedt, Professor at Copenhagen, concerning the action of a galvanic current on a magnetized needle,

[1] Loridan, op. cit., p. 159.

I have thought about it continually ; I have done nothing
but write a great theory concerning these phenomena,
and all others known about magnets, and try experiments
indicated by this theory, all of which have been successful
and have taught me a large number of new facts. I read
the beginning of a paper at the meeting of the Institute
a week ago to-day. On the following days I made
confirmative experiments, partly with Fresnel, and
partly with Desprets. I repeated them all on Friday
evening at Poisson's, where there was a partly consisting
of the two Mussys, Rendu, several pupils of the École
Normale, General Campredon, etc. Everything succeeded
marvellously ; but the decisive experiment, which I had
conceived as definite proof, needed two galvanic batteries.
When it was tried with batteries which were too weak at
Fresnel's, it did not succeed. Yesterday, however,
I at last obtained Dulong's permission to Dumotier to
sell me the large battery which he was having built for
the physics course of the Faculty, and which had just been
finished. This morning, the experiment was made at
Dumotier's with complete success, and repeated to-day
at four o'clock at the meeting of the Institute. No
further objections were put to me, and we have a new
theory of the magnet which relates all the phenomena
to those of galvanism."

Ampère was not alone in his invention. Just as in
repeating Oerstedt's experiment, he saw by intuition the
identity between the magnet and the current, so he utilized
Laplace's ideas. The latter suggested to him an
experiment concerning the displacement of a magnetized
needle at a great distance by means of a current. Ampère
immediately deduced from this the first project for an
electric telegraph. He mentions it in his Memoir of the
2nd October, 1820. " By means of as many conducting
wires and magnetized needles as there are letters, and
by placing each letter on a different needle, one might
establish the action of a battery placed a long way from
these needles and able to be connected to any one of the

wires, on any of the needles, and so make a sort of *telegraph* capable of writing any news which it was desired to transmit, pass no matter what obstacles to the person charged with observing the letters placed on the needles, by arranging a keyboard on the battery, the key of which would be marked with the same letters and would establish communication by being pressed down, this means of communication could be made quite easy, and would take no longer than the time necessary to touch the key at one end and read the letters at the other." [1]

The telegraph was envisaged by a flash of intuition, resulting from latent reasoning, which is partly unconscious. Ampère for two months made numerous conscious researches with the object of realizing the telegraph. "All this winter of 1820 to 1821," says M. de Launay, "he had no other idea than this in his head ; sensational communications followed one another on the 9th, 16th, 30th of October, the 6th, 13th and 27th November, the 4th, 11th and 26th of December."

At this moment Arago came to the help of Ampère : "On the 10th November, 1820, Arago conceived the idea of plunging into iron filings a wire traversed by a current. If, as Ampère's theory requires, galvanism and magnetism are identical, the iron filings will be attracted as they would be by a magnet. It was in fact so."

Arago showed this experiment to Ampère. The latter immediately drew this deduction from it : If a needle of soft iron is placed in a current having a spiral path, it would be turned into a temporary magnet. "The experiment, which Ampère and Arago successfully performed together, produced the electro-magnet." [2]

Arago, in his first experiment, had thus demonstrated a fact, but had not drawn the conclusion ; Ampère immediately saw the more distant conclusion, before performing an experiment, by a sort of logical anticipation.

[1] De Launay, op. cit., pp. 196, 197, 198.
[2] Op. cit., p. 198.

This experiment succeeded and served as a proof for Arago and as a verification for Ampère.

Let us define, from the psychological point of view, the work in Ampère's mind which resulted in the invention of electro-dynamics.

(1) His character, his precocious scientific studies constitute a distant preparation for his great discoveries ; a *conscious* preparation relatively to the studies to which he directly devoted himself, an unconscious preparation relatively to future inventions, for he was not yet thinking of them.

(2) These inventions came into being as a result of collaboration with other physicists, Oerstedt, Laplace, Arago. These furnished him with experiments which served as points of departure ; they prepared the way for him ; they cleared and built the road into the experimental domain. They stated the major premise of a syllogism, but did not draw the conclusion. This conclusion was seen suddenly by Ampère, namely, that it was a matter of identifying a magnet and a current, or that the electro-magnet, and hence electric telegraphy, were possible. The conclusion was foreseen with certainty, before the minor of the experiment allowed him to generalize ; and that is why the famous physicist once in possession of his fertile idea, could not rest before he saw a complete demonstration of it. For the same reason he made numerous experiments, sure of the result, uneasy only on the subject of the method. All this verification, a minor of the syllogism, was fully conscious.

We thus return to the theory of the unconscious as a process of reasoning where one proposition is half understood. This unconscious, as we have seen, is partial. The conclusion comes about so quickly because the mind glides rapidly over the minor of the syllogism. But the minor, being still a hypothesis, was in need of proof. That is why the premature conclusion is followed by a luxuriant crop of experimental demonstration.

Such is the very limited part which we think should be assigned to the unconscious in these physical inventions of Ampère.

7. *A Chemical Invention—The Match*

In passing from physics to chemistry, we still continue to find that experiment plays a preponderating part in inventions. Let us consider the discovery which allowed us to give up the use of the flint for obtaining fire. The inventor of matches, Charles Sauria, was born at Poligny in 1812. His father wished him to become a doctor, and he had obtained the title of Doctor at the Faculty of Besançon. He practised at Saint-Lathain, a hamlet in the Jura, where he died in 1895. The following are the circumstances under which he was led to produce the invention which remained his masterpiece.

"While on a journey to Lyons in 1827, young Sauria was very much intrigued by seeing a hydrogen lighter which an optician had placed at the entrance of his shop. This "hydroplatinic lamp", as it was called, had just been invented by Gay-Lussac; but being difficult to carry about it was only a very imperfect solution of the problem of producing domestic fire.

Also, on returning to College at Dole, he was haunted by the idea of discovering a more convenient method of making a light, and set to work. He sought for a fulminating powder which would allow him to realize his dream. In December, 1830, Nicolet, his Professor of chemistry, repeated an experiment which struck him; it was the well-known experiment which consists in causing in a mortar, by means of a light blow, the detonation of a powdered mixture of sulphur and chlorate of potash. He suddenly thought that if one could incorporate a mixture of these two substances with phosphorus, one would obtain fire. His sagacity was not at fault.

"Alas, Sauria's means of conducting his researches

were very limited, and his inexperience in manipulation hindered him greatly. Tubes were broken, he often burnt his hands. Once, even the curtains of his bed caught fire, but the little strips of wood did not catch fire. Finally our philosopher pupil had the idea of dipping the extremity of the sulphur-coated wood into heated chlorate, and a few particles of chlorate stuck to the sulphur. Sauria was rewarded for his persevering labour, for the match was no sooner prepared than when rubbed on the wall, on which were traces of phosphorus, it caught fire at once.

" A short time afterwards the young inventor perfected his discovery. He added gum arabic in order to make the mixture of chlorate of potash, sulphur and phosphorus adhere better to the wood.[1]

Considering the various circumstances in which this invention was brought about, we come to the following conclusion. First of all, he was inspired by a lively *desire*. Sauria had seen a hydrogen lighter, which was not a very practical instrument. He sought for a better one. The apparatus suggested by Gay-Lussac was, however, a first solution of the problem. Its defect is that of lighting with difficulty. But seeing it, suggested to Sauria the idea of the fulminating powder which could produce light instantaneously. He thought of it from that day onward. He never ceased to work at it from the time of his return to College : a ferment of ideas the conscious course of which could not be perceived, was produced in his young intelligence.

But it was here that his Professor of chemistry, two months afterwards, came to his aid by the experiment made with chlorate of potash and sulphur. The explosion in this case is a realization of the rapid production of fire. Sulphur and chlorate of potash are therefore capable of producing it. The conclusion immediately flashes before the eyes of the patient seeker. " He thought of it immediately," said the author of the account. It was a

[1] Boyer; article in the *Echo de Paris*, 1st March, 1925.

subjective certainty for him, but there was not yet any evidence for all the world, since the experiment had not been made. Before this experiment, in this divination of the right procedure to be followed, there were still traces of the unconscious; for only a rapid induction could have confered this certainty upon him ; and we have seen that induction, anticipated generalization, cannot be produced without logical intermediaries which are taken for granted.

We then have conscious attempts. Sauria tried, burnt himself and started again : his efforts were in vain.

But one day the idea came to him of dipping the sulphur of the match into heated chlorate. This was the decisive inspiration ; the procedure proved successful. Where did this idea come from ? Doubtless from the successful results already furnished by the association of sulphur and chlorate. But the young man only thought of it after numerous failures ; it had thus remained in his mind as a possibility held in reserve, without his knowing it. It was the need for success which caused this ingenious combination to pass from the potential to the actual.

Thus at two different stages in the history of this invention, unconscious work preceded conscious experiment ; the latter being nothing but the verification of the correctness of the procedure which the author had glimpsed and which appeared to him certain of success since he worked without ceasing to demonstrate it.

8. *The Invention of a Science by means of the Apparatus of Physics*

The inventions of physical science pave the way for other inventions. The Abbé Rousselot offers us a characteristic example. In his case, the prodution of a new apparatus enabled him to elaborate a theory and create a new science, experimental phonetics.

(a) The distant preparation

He was born at Saint-Claude in Charente, and from his childhood he listened with great attention to the original speech of his country. As a Professor he had a taste for etymology, and studied particularly the transformation which words suffer when passing from father to son, and from one country to another. He was particularly interested in the inquiry undertaken in 1873 by MM. Bringuier and Tourtoulers for the purpose of fixing the geographical limits of the *langue d'oïl* and the *langue d'oc*. These researches proved to him the insufficiency of linguistic methods.

(b) Nearer preparation

Wishing to introduce more precision into this science, he came to Paris in 1880, studied linguistics there, also comparative grammar, physiology, and the physical sciences, with Paul Meyer, Gaston Paris, Edouard Branly, Becquerel and Marey, who was the inventor of an apparatus for registering the vibratory movements of the larynx. The society of these scientists stimulated his taste for research.

(c) The first invention ; Apparatus

He then also became an inventor on his own account of more delicate instruments : the electric membrane recorder, the pneumograph, and the artificial palate. These pieces of apparatus, constructed as a result of his knowledge of physical science, allowed him to create a new science.

(d) Second invention : Experimental phonetics

When Professor at the Catholic Institute at Paris, he prepared a thesis for his Doctorate entitled *Modifications in Language in a family of Cellefrouin*, a place near his birthplace. Thanks to a laboratory set up at his request at the College de France, he continued to experiment and published in 1908 his *Principles of*

Experimental Phonetics. The War of 1914 allowed him to verify his theory. He made use of his knowledge of acoustics to find the position of enemy batteries.

Thus, experimental phonetics was created. It has its principles ; it has been verified. Its inventor, who, as his biographer says, " has always kept in his researches the joy and certitude of resolving the problems undertaken," was nominated, in 1922, Professor of Experimental Phonetics at the Collège de France.

Three facts must be kept in mind.

(1) Distant preparation was unconscious. The scientist to be hears the peasants talking, seeks for etymologies, follows a scientific quest ; but this was because he had a taste for these things and a desire to know about them, without any known relation to his inventions as a Professor

(2) On the other hand, the fusion of the natural sciences, the physical sciences and linguistics, was accomplished consciously in his mind ; he knows what his aim is, he can foresee the end, the possibility of a new science based on the result of sciences already studied.

(3) His invention was realized ; it is a double one. The first consists in machines constructed analagously to the apparatus of Branly, Marey, etc. We find here the unconscious element inherent in all analogical syntheses. The second is the science itself, experimental phonetics. When once the principles have been stated as a result of concordant experiments, the edifice is built logically and consciously on its foundations. There we have no sudden inspiration, no revelation half seen in a flash. The whole is produced in the clear light of reason, but for the mysterious work of synthetic connection which, following Dwelshauvers, we have called the rational unconscious.

9. Conclusion

The place which we must assign to reflection in conscious work in this branch of science is considerable. This

I

preponderance is necessary. How, indeed, could one observe without full attention being given ? What would be the use of experiment, which is observation of set purpose, if it is not commenced and conducted by a mind ceaselessly awake to retain suggestive details ?

It is easy to define the field in which unconscious preparation operates, however small the part it plays, by summarizing what we have found from the preceding examples.

(1) When we investigate the origin of all work directed towards the production of an invention, we find a lively *desire*, sometimes even an imperious *need*, and what is almost a *passion* for success. It was with the object of eliminating from science an absurd cause—"nature abhors a vacuum "—that Galilei, Torricelli, and Pascal performed their experiments upon atmospheric pressure. It was because they desired to fix luminous images that Wedgewood, Davy, Charles, Nicéphore Niepce and Daguerre tried the many experiments which resulted in photography. Foucault wished to demonstrate the rotation of the earth, and he divined the measure of a very small angle which he had to use for supporting his proof. Having learned of Oerstedt's experiment Ampère was filled with eagerness to exploit it, and could not rest until he had established, together with Arago, the solid foundations of electro-dynamics. Sauria noticed the defects of the hydrogen lighter and "hydro-platinic lamp " invented by Gay Lussac, and we see in experimenting, haunted by the idea of discovering a more practical method of making fire. It is this ardent desire of realizing something still only vaguely defined which supports inventors in their numerous trials, however varied and often even unfruitful these may be.

(2) In the case of all inventors and all constructors of systems, *conscious* preparation is long and varied. Newton studied the researches of Galilei and Huyghens on weight before developing his theory of universal attraction. Torricelli and Pascal had read Aristotle,

Bacon, and Galilei. Feeling the same horror of a vacuum as nature herself, they discovered atmospheric pressure behind this metaphysical phantom, and the invention of the barometer, followed by that of the manometer was the fruit of long preliminary study. In the same way, Daguerre's print was preceded by numerous trials from 1799 to 1830 ; Watt and Wedgewood prepared the way for Niepce and Daguerre. Turning to the cinematograph, the brothers Auguste and Louis Lumiere were acquainted with the previous attempts of Marey. The law of double refraction given by Fresnel and Huyghens inspired Malus the inventor of the repeating goniometer. Foucault studied mathematics in order to invent in physics. Ampère acquired enclyclopædic knowledge before devising the principle of the telegraph. Rousselot studied physics before creating experimental phonetics. Sauria only invented matches after having experimented with the effects of chlorate of potassium. Enthusiastic and often very long study, considered utilization of the work of numerous predecessors, research done in collaboration with several contemporaries ; such is the conscious activity which we find as the *substratum* of inventive work.

(3) Let us now consider the decisive moment at which the fundamental idea is revealed, the elaboration of which has been unconscious, in some degree however small. In Newton's case, sitting under his apple tree, it was a flash of identification between solar and terrestrial attraction ; the work which had preceded this sudden analogy had been unconscious. Without thinking about it, Torricelli made use of a barometer when he wished to test the pressure of the atmosphere ; there was an element of the unconscious in his attempt. There was nothing of the kind in the experiment by which Pascal extended and generalized Torricelli's discovery. Niepce's fertile idea consisted in the discovery of a remarkable property of asphaltum. In Daguerre's case it was the perception of the connection between the existence of

mercury vapour and the appearance of the image on a photographic plate ; this glimpse of a causal connection was a surprise, but unconscious labour had preceded ti. In the case of the cinematograph, we are not conscious of the actual discontinuity of the pictures thrown on the screen ; the inventor's originality consisted in realizing before experience had proved it that the rapid succession of discontinuous images would give the illusion of continuity. Without thinking about it, Malus turned his prism between his fingers ; and, after performing this movement unconsciously, he suddenly formulated his hypothesis on the polarization of light. Foucault had an intuition of the value of an angle before Bertrand made his calculation ; this divination was the result of unconscious thinking. The same anticipation took place in Ampère's mind ; he identified the magnet with a current as soon as he knew of Oerstedt's experiment ; this sudden conclusion was the logical result of implied reasoning.

The inventor of matches sprang over the logical step in the same manner ; his professor had demonstrated the detonation of a mixture of sulphur and chlorate. Sauria immediately thought of mixing phosporus with these two substances. This was the fertile idea, and also a hasty conclusion since the decisive experiments were still to be made ; thus unconscious work had caused this idea to spring into his mind. It is thus certain when we consider all the facts, that the fundamental idea of the invention seems to hatch out suddenly after some experimental groping preceded by a long conscious preparation. Now, on the one hand, the first experiments are not sufficient to justify the generality of the conclusion. On the other hand, the preceding conscious study bears indirectly on the essential object of the invention. Thus an internal labour is necessary to choose in these studies the necessary elements for the invention, and to justify the sudden inspiration, which is like a crystallization of this synthesis. But this elaboration is partly unconscious, since the conclusion springs up before the experimental premises have been consciously set forth. Thus the traces of the unconscious which we discover in this mental labour have preceded an anticipated conclusion. This conclusion is the fundamental idea of the invention.

(4) We then have, following on this flash of identification, a new period of conscious activity. The mind, delighted to have glimpsed the end, cannot be satisfied until it has illuminated the road which it appears to have passed over like a bird in flight. This is the phase of experimental verification, of the justification which is necessary for the hypothesis.

This time is necessarily long, for, on the one hand, the unconscious has only prepared a hypothetical conclusion which must be confirmed by facts, and, on the other hand, this experimental confirmation requires, if it is not to be faulty, a very varied series of proofs and counter proofs, without which the conclusion would not be scientifically general.

Newton verified his theory in two stages separated by an interval of four years, first with an erroneous value for the meridian, afterwards with a correct one. Torricelli's beautiful experiment was confirmed by Pascal and his brother-in-law Périer, in two places, at the Puy-de-Dome and at Paris. Further confirmation was given by the constructors of various barometers and manometers. Niepce, and above all Daguerre, prepared a piece of conscious verification which Talbot, Nicéphore Niepce assisted by his cousin Victor, and Professor Korn continued. In the same way, when once they had conceived the first idea, the brothers Lumière created the cinema by a series of inventions, improvements, and successive modification. Also conscious were the repeated experiments of Malus for verifying the polarization of light, those of Ampère, with the help of Poisson, Fresnel, and Arago, for founding electro-dynamics and inventing the electric telegraph. Take Sauria : Once he had dreamed of a better means of obtaining fire than the hydroplatinic lamp, and knowing the detonating power of chlorate of potash, he made numerous experiments with chlorate alone, then with chlorate mixed with sulphur and phosphorus.

We see from all these examples that the unconscious work of the inventor was, in most cases, the latent fermentation of results acquired in preceding, fully conscious, work. This caused a fertile idea, the hypothesis, the foreseen conclusion, to spring into the mind, to be verified afterwards by quite deliberate experiments. As in the case of the mathematical sciences, but with less precision and suddenness, the invention was revealed quite suddenly after hidden incubation, preceded by a luminous phase and followed by a second phase of clarity. In certain cases, such as Volta and Branly the idea of the battery and the idea of wireless telegraphy were the logical results of profound meditation and long experiment. In their cases as in many others, so they tell us, there was nothing unforeseen ; it would be rash to introduce into their . researches a period of unconsciousness. The imporant properties of matter with which the physical sciences are concerned, can only be discovered by vigorous workers who devote patient labour and reflection to this purpose. In their generality, these properties are perceived by a sort of metaphysic based upon experience. We know the series of calculations which these sciences imply and what a large part is to be given to observation. Now observation assumes attention, and hence consciousness. Thus the field of the unforeseen, the domain of sudden discoveries, is necessarily restricted. It exists nevertheless.

CHAPTER IV

THE UNCONSCIOUS AND INVENTION IN THE BIOLOGICAL SCIENCES

The place of the unconscious in these sciences—The theorists : Le Dantec, Cuvier, Oscar Schmidt, Grasset, Claude Bernard — The unconscious in the case of the experimenters—Claude Bernard, Haüy—Louis Pasteur : theory and practice—Darwin and his evolutionary hypothesis—Conclusion.

I. THE POSSIBLE PLACE OF THE UNCONSCIOUS IN THESE SCIENCES

BY the term *biological sciences* we here understand zoology, botany, geology, and palæontology. They have also been grouped by M. Goblot under the term physiology, the science of the functions of living beings.[1]

We may remark to begin with, that life is the new factor which differentiates these sciences from those of physics and chemistry. Now life manifests itself with infinite variety in the animal and vegetable world. In order to study living beings scientifically it is necessary to disentangle from the mobility and variability of forms, certain essential characters, and distinguish them from accidental characters ; and, if they are dominant characters, to separate them from characters which are subordinate to them. Fundamentally, the sciences of living beings consider the relations of constant simultaneity between them. In order to establish these, we proceed by analogy and by hypothesis, in order to arrive finally at classification and definition.

[1] Goblot, *Le système des sciences*, ix, pp. 101–43.

Also, as in the case of physics and chemistry, it is necessary, before undertaking experiments, to be in possession of a " directing idea," for otherwise our direction would be left to chance. This idea may appear suddenly, like a flash, or after a long period of preparation. In both cases, its birth is unforeseen. On the other hand, the experiments themselves are most frequently initiated by an observation made in a previous experiment, sometimes even by an impression to which the scientist has paid little attention. He thus is experimenting haphazardly.

We find, then, traces of the unconscious in the suggestion of the fertile idea and in the personal inspiration which directs the scientist in his experimenting.

The foregoing is what we can state *a priori* from the actual nature of the biological sciences. We may now hear the reasoned opinion of the scientists, who, in this field, may be considered in some cases as theoriticians, in some cases as experimenters concerning the psychological conditions of invention.

THE THEORISTS OF INVENTION

1.   Le Dantec, and his Interpretation of the Laws of Chance

Le Dantec gives us an explanation of chance which is sufficiently curious to be noted ; it will give us the opportunity of defining the various cases in which the unconscious finds its place in explaining events.

(1) " There is chance when an unforseen event happens to an animal : Chance is *the unforeseen*."

(2) " There is chance when we know the general lines of a future phenomenon, but not the detail itself. Chance is the *unforeseeable*."

(3) " There is chance, if we know the laws of phenomena, but not the precise data which allow us to

draw conclusions from them. Chance is the *unexpected conclusion*."

(4) " There is chance if we know the law, but do not know the data of the particular case. Chance is the *particular case*."

(5) " There is chance for everyone, if the phenomena do not obey any law. Chance is the *absence of any law*."

But Le Dantec, who is a determinist, cannot accept these definitions which he feels obliged to formulate with implacable logic. The pretended laws of chance, admitted by H. Poincaré, Bernoulli, and so many others, are thus rejected by him.

He concludes : " What Poincaré calls ' the law of chance ' is the certainty that the phenomena do not obey any law," which is inadmissible from the scientific point of view.[1]

We think, with Le Dantec, that chance, defined as he understands it is absurd. It would be, in fact, the suppression of universal causality, and, consequently, it would imply the impossibility of science. But the reasoning is fanciful. The word chance is not devoid of sense. It signifies for the common man every unexpected, unforeseen, and even unforeseeable event. In this respect Le Dantec is right. But who denies the existence of a cause of which he is ignorant ? Is to avow one's ignorance, to deny science ? Is the unforeseen non-existent ? M. Souriau, whose views on inventions we shall describe at length later on, defines chance more successfully than Le Dantec, as " the conflict between external and internal finality ". His thought is as follows : externally to ourselves, universal determinism insists that every effect will be logically connected with its cause. On the other hand, in our minds, the psychological mechanism of the association of ideas necessarily produces a mental synthesis by virtue of internal determinism. Now let a fact astonish us ; our astonish-

---

[1] Le Dantec, *Le chaos et l'harmonie universelle*, Paris, 1911, pp. 87 et 105.

ment arises from the disagreement between the form in which the new event is clothed, and the aspect which our internal logic has to attribute to it.   We qualify the event as fortuitous, but instead of denying chance as does Le Dantec, we give it a rational interpretation.   As being a conflict between our judgment and the external fact, chance implies a double ignorance which may be a double unconsciousness: the unconsciousness of the relation which exists between an effect and a cause—which we may know perhaps, but do not think of—the unconsciousness born of the absolute ignorance of the cause. Here we are interested only in the first form.   In the case of experiments performed by scientists, the surprise caused by chance may often be the prelude to a revelation.   The consciousness, being obliged to note the surprising character of the fact, is in some respects behind the unconscious, which is already possessed of a certainty which will soon appear in full daylight.   Thus, to put it more precisely, chance is nothing but a delay imposed on conscious logic.

2. Cuvier and his Vocation as a Naturalist

Let us consider Cuvier.   When Permanent Secretary of the Academy of Sciences, he was the author of the celebrated theory of the *laws of finality*, the foundation of generalization in natural history.   He formulated this principle as follows : " Since nothing can exist unless it comprises the conditions which make its existence possible, the different parts of every being must be co-ordinated in such a manner as to render the whole being possible not only in itself, but also in its relations with those which surround it."[1]

" As a child, he read a copy of Buffon ; he copied the pictures of the animals ; they inspired him with

---

[1] Cuvier, *Regne animal*, introduction, p. 8.

the taste for natural history and description . . . At
Stuttgart, he read Linnæus, he read him for ten years.
. . . When a teacher in Normandy he saw terebratulæ,
and compared the fossils with living species ; he dissected
molluscs . . . He discovered four general forms of
the nervous system."

Later on, he conceived the method of recognizing each
bone and distinguishing it from every other with
certainty ; he assigned each bone to the species to which
it belonged ; he finally reconstructed the complete
skeleton of each species, without omitting any piece
proper to it, and without inserting any piece which did
not belong to it.

The idea of the general plan of the world of animals
had thus been inspired in him by the intellectual
experience of his adolescence. His theory had been
suggested to him little by little by the unconscious,
which we might call here the unconscious of education.

3. *Oscar Schmidt: The Unconscious in the Biological
Sciences*

Cuvier was a creator. Oscar Schmidt was merely
the commentator on Hartmann's doctrine of the
unconscious as applied to the natural sciences. His
statement is none the less interesting.

He remarks, first of all, that in this respect Hartmann
borrowed part of his ideas, Carus, the Dresden
philosopher. These ideas are as follows.

We know the importance of the principle of purpose
in biology. Now " the teleological idea "—that is to say
the concept of purpose—is of capital importance in the
philosophy of the unconscious.[1]

Hartmann, in fact, holds that " the unconscious is a
spiritus rector ". It is what drives the bee to construct
the hexagonal cells of its comb, what causes the special

[1] Oscar Schmidt, *Les sciences naturelles et la philosophie de
l'inconscient*, Paris, 1879, p. 4.

instinct of certain dogs to develop, and also what, in the vegetable world, sets the wind and the insects to work to ensure the fertilization of flowers. Fundamentally, the unconscious is the generic terms which designates what the metaphysicians call " final causes ".

If this is the case, what relation must be established between the consciousness and the unconsciousness ? How are they to be diagnosed ? Where does one begin and the other end ? " The consciousness is the emancipation of the idea with respect to the will, while they are both, idea and will, indissolubly united in the unconscious. The unconscious is ' the unconscious soul of the world '. It is a little like the God of the Theists." [1]

If we introduce a little French clarity into these nebulous remarks of the German metaphysician, as regards the idea and the will, two distinct moments : 1. The idea is united to the will, and it is impossible to distinguish them. This is the *unconscious* phase ; it is an idea animated by the will, it is an idea which is ignorant of itself, it is a blind thrust. This is certainly true of animal instincts and the natural tendencies of vegetables. 2. We pass farther up the scale ; the idea is no longer subjected to the will, it has emancipated itself from its tutelage. Having become adult in some way, it is independent. But now it is no longer a blind instinct, it has become *consciousness*.

In the case of Man, regarded as an animal very much higher than the others, the unconscious and the consciousness are not two successive stages, they do not represent two incompatible concepts. They are rather, in the human soul, two distinct plans, which collaborate in all forms of activity. Now, in the case of the animals and plants, the unconscious, analagous to the " finality " of metaphysicians and the " function " of modern scientists—drives the living being to organize what is necessary for itself. Is not this a kind of invention ? In the case of Man, likewise, the unconscious works

[1] Op. cit., p. 112.

cunningly at a discovery, but—and, in this respect, Man is much superior to other living beings—the unconscious is quickly joined in this creative work by the consciousness. Thus, in the case of Man, the two plans of inventive activity reunite, at a given moment, to reinforce one-another.

Such is the original theory of Hartmann as expounded by Oscar Schmidt. It shows—while placing Man in the animal series—in what an admirable fashion his invention surpasses the instinctive production of inferior living creatures.

4. *Grasset and his Theory of two Psychisms*

Grasset's theory of the " two psychisms " is still more interesting. If we develop it here it is because it is at once psychological and physiological. What we call consciousness is for him the *superior* psychism ; what we call the relatively unconscious is for him the *inferior* psychism or the *polygon*. First of all, he defines the sense of the world psychism. It is not the occult. It is not necessarily the consciousness. For the acts of the lower psychism are psychical and nevertheless, they are at least partially unconscious. It is every phenomenon in which there is thought, intelligence in any degree. While the consciousness, for him, is without degree, is always the clear consciousness of the psychologists, the psychism admits of a large variety of degrees : it will be *superior*, if the conscienciousness is clear ; it is *inferior* in every other case.

We must thus note that the term psychism means any intellectual activity whatsoever, while in this palace of the mind, consciousness only represents those floors which are illuminated.

This being stated the adjoining figure explains sufficiently well Grasset's conceptions of the two psychisms.

The centre O represents the superior psychism,

consciousness. It is here that the various neurones converge. Consciousness exists if communication is established. If it fails there is disaggregation.

The remainder of the figure, EMKAVT, is the inferior psychism, or polygon. A represents the auditory centre, V the visual, T the tactile (the sensorial centre), K the kinematic, M speech, E writing (motor centres). Without entering into any more detail we can easily conceive that clear consciousness may exist if the various centres are connected with the centre O. Now suppose that the connections of the various centres with O are broken, but their connections with one another remain, or at least those of some of them with

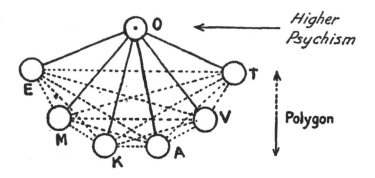

their neighbours. There is no longer consciousness, since O no longer receives the sensations of the neurones, but there is always an interpolygonal activity which remains, and this is that of inferior psychism. In this region " there is the possibility of will and attention, but automatism and unconsciousness ".

By automatism Grasset understands " an activity which is apparently spontaneous but without free will "

The following is the polygonal theory of inspiration. The author adopts the ideas of Chabaneix and de Regis : " there are individuals who show at certain moments, sometimes during the day, sometimes at night, a peculiar state between sleeping and waking, between consciousness and unconsciousness. The personality of men of talent and genius is rather made up of nervous erethism than of madness ; great creators are not insane ; they are waking sleepers who are lost in their unconscious abstraction, beings apart who walk, living in their starry dream."

Grasset also adopts this explanation of Ribot's : " inspiration resembles a cipher despatch transmitted by unconscious activity to conscious activity, which translates it. The richness of the invention depends upon the subliminal imagination, not upon the other, which is superficial by nature and quickly exhausted. Inspiration is a sign of unconscious imagination. Psychologically, this state is produced by various attitudes which augment the circulation : walking with long strides, or on the contrary, lying stretched out ; darkness is sought, or on the contrary a bright light ; the feet are put in' water or in ice, the head in full sunshine ; use is made of wine, spirits, aromatic drinks, haschich, etc."

The two psychical centres collaborate in inspiration ; the combination is at once conscious and unconscious, the result is harmonious.

The author gives a number of examples which corroborate his theory.

Walter Scott went to bed after having confided to the inferior polygon an idea to be expressed or developed. On waking up he found the expression sought for.

According to Rémy de Gourmont, " the consciousness is not the principle of art : far from being united to the functioning of the consciousness, intellectual activity is more often deranged by it. We think badly when we know that we are thinking. Intellectual and imaginative creation is inseparable from the frequent occurence of a sub-conscious condition." [1]

Burdach, the Konigsberg professor, made several

---

[1] Rémy de Gourmont: *La création subconsciente.* Paris, 1900, p. 47.

physical discoveries while dreaming, which he was afterwards able to verify. A dream was the point of departure for a work. It is probable that conscious reasoning, on awakening, rectified the dream and gave it its true value.

Goethe believed that all talent implies an instinctive force acting in the unconscious.

Finally, according to Grasset, it was certainly with the superior psychism O that Newton, Claude Bernard, and Pasteur made their discoveries. They nevertheless worked on the products of the polygon.

The role of the conscious psychism is to initiate, direct, and revitalize the polygon. It is the creative genius. But it is the polygon's task to ruminate and develop. In a sense, " the power of comparing, of reasoning, of judging, belongs to all psychic centres, to the inferior as well as to the superior. But the general laws of logic are but ill-observed by them ; reasoning is illogical and superficial, as we see in hypnosis."

If we recall the diagram showing the relations of the neurones with one another and with the centre O we can understand this discontinuity in the mechanism of reasoning. Nevertheless, does not Grasset confuse the association of ideas with truly rational operations ? We will discuss this question in the second part of this study.

For the moment, we may remark that this psychological theory appears to be corroborated by phenomena which occur at the commencement of sleep. For instance, one has been engaged upon the investigation of a certain question. In the state of complete wakefulness all considerations suggested by the fundamental idea appeared to gravitate regularly around the latter, as a true centre of connection, while preserving points of attachment to neighbouring ideas. One now commences to fall asleep : the ideas diverge little by little ; they lose all contact with the directive centre ; however, if they are compared with the secondary ideas likewise originally nourished by the same original idea, they preserve their first cohesion with the latter.

For my part, I have confirmed this when giving a mathematics lecture during the War. As an over-tired soldier, I heard the replies of my pupil while half asleep. At first, my explanations, which were a continuation of his, always related to the theorem which was to be proved. But, having by chance alluded to the arrangement of soldiers in a battle in order to show the pupil the method of arranging proofs in view of a conclusion, I soon forgot, while half asleep, the demonstration itself, and occasionally, in replying to the pupil, I spoke of events of the War. Obviously, the conscious centre O had been put out of the discussion, while the neurones of the polygon continued their normal activity and associated ideas relating to the war.

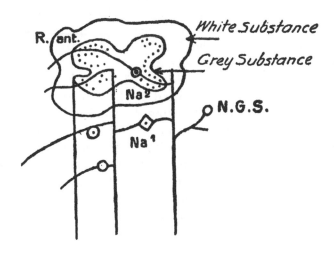

We may attach this unconscious polygonal activity to that of the spinal cord, which is always unconscious. The internal prolongation of the afferent neurone of the spinal ganglion N.G.S. penetrates into the white substance : it divides into two branches : the descending branch goes to join the efferent neurone on the same side ; the ascending branch passes upwards to the medulla to branch out in the grey matter. These branches are joined to efferent neurones through the neurones of association ; of these latter, those such as Na^1 are directed towards the same side of the cord, the others, Na^2, to the opposite side. Thus the nervous impulse transmitted by the centripetal N.G.S. is connected to several efferent neurones N.C. It expands, *irradiates*. However, in this case, these neurones have no connection with the conscious centre O.

This unconscious mechanism, which is normal when it takes place in the spinal cord, is intermittent during sleep. But this *irradiation* of the neurones is then more general ; it has for its field the whole of the nervous centres. Since, during sleep, the nervous termini are somewhat disconnected among themselves, unconsciousness is explained because all relation has been broken with the centre O. But by means of irradiation of the secondary neurone and the neurones of association, we can account for the fact that the activity of the unconscious polygon is permanent.

We may generalize this idea. That which is constant in the spinal cord, but limited to the zone of this cord, that which is intermittent during sleep and extended to the majority of nervous zones, may surely exist at all times, in some degree, in the totality of the nervous system. Under these conditions, the centre O is apprized of the activity of the centres in relation with it, and we have consciousness, but a limited consciousness. On the other hand, there is a considerable region whose connection with O is not regular. In this quasi-autonomous psychical region, the unconscious affects all the transformations and developments which will one day be submitted later to the control of the conscious metropolis.[1]

---

[1] Cf. Wâustier, *Sciences naturelles à l'usage des classes de philosophie et de mathématiques*, Paris, 1923, pp. 296–8.

5. *Claude Bernard and his theory of the relation between the consciousness and the unconscious*

Claude Bernard, who has given a theory of discoveries and inventions in biology, has put forward a view concerning the relationship between the unconscious and discovery or invention which deserves to become classical.

First of all, what is *discovery* ? It is " the new idea which arises in connection with a fact found by chance or otherwise ". Hence in discovery itself there is, by definition, this unforeseen thing, this unexpected event, this fortuitous case which presupposes unconsciousness in its antecedents. The fact is conscious, its preparation is either conscious or unconscious.

It follows from this " that we can make two kinds of discoveries in the sciences. One kind is foreseen by reason or indicated by theory. It presupposes two conditions : a highly advanced science, physics for example, and simple phenomena. The other kind is unforeseen. They arise unexpectedly during experiment not as corollaries of theory and adapted to confirm the latter, but always outside of it, and hence opposed to it ".

Now the discovery, that is to say, the new idea found by chance, very often can only become a law if it explains a collection of facts, if it is the expression of a uniformity in nature, or in other words, a constant relationship between phenomena. Hence two conditions are necessary in order that discovery or invention may be possible : (1) Determinism in nature, without which there would be no constancy in the phenomena reproduced and hence no possibility of law. (2) Freedom of mind, that is to say, the intellectual disposition through which a scientist is always ready to abandon a previous theory in the presence of new facts which show it to be false or even uncertain in character. Hence, no fixed ideas : " those who have an excessive faith in their ideas are ill suited to making discoveries."[1] Thus, from the psychological point of view, it may happen that contrary to all preconceived ideas, the fundamental idea of the discovery or invention may be formed suddenly without a conscious basis to justify it.

What is therefore the genesis of this fertile idea which not being produced by another one, seems to be an absolute beginning ? Claude Bernard, like H. Poincaré, sees the source of it in a pre-existent feeling : " feeling always takes the initiative ; it engenders the *a priori* idea or the intuition." The order of phenomena is vaguely felt ; this feeling arouses the idea of a first experiment in which certain details produce a new feeling generating a new idea. The second idea calls in its turn the confirmation by a second experiment, and so on. Now this succession of feelings and ideas remains vague ; the mind passes through them without noticing the scarcely perceptible transitions. That is why Bernard sees in it a form of reasoning :—

" Experimental and relative reasoning is external and unconscious." On the other hand, as Goethe, quoted by Claude Bernard, remarked, " Experiment is the sole mediator between the objective and the subjective, that is to say, between phenomena and the sciences." Experiment is thus absolutely necessary, and since the succession of ideas and feelings which it presupposes contains unconscious elements, the unconscious has a necessary place in experimental reasoning.

Hence, by experimenting, " man becomes an inventor of phenomena, a true foreman of creation ; he submits his idea to nature." But since each experiment calls for its successor by the details which it brings to our notice, " the greatest scientific truths have their roots in the details of experimental investigations " ; consequently, " these details are as it were the soil in which they are developed."

[1] Claude Bernard, *Leçons de physiologie expérimentale appliquée à la médicine, faites au Collège de France*, Paris, 1885, pp. 17–67.

Is there therefore a method for discovering an invention? What part does it play ?

" There is no method for making discoveries. Philosophical theories cannot give the feeling for invention to those who do not know it." Rather, " A bad method may stifle the genius for invention, but a good method develops it."

On the other hand, " the idea, that *quid proprium* which constitutes originality, the invention or genius of anyone, only develops in surroundings which predispose the mind to it." Hence it follows that the same ideas are found among individuals at a like level. Simultaneous inventions are therefore possible. Further, " in experimental methods, every great man belongs to his time, and can only come at his right moment. For there is a necessary and subordinate succession in scientific discoveries." We thus find here, as in mathematical and physical sciences, a collaboration, partly unconscious and partly conscious, in discovery and invention ; " it most often happens that, in the evolution of science, the various parts of experimental reasoning are shared by several men."

Finally, Claude Bernard generalizes and distinguishes as follows the two phases of the unconscious and the consciousness in scientific work :—

" There is a kind of instruction or unconscious experience which is obtained by the practice of something. . . . Experience may be acquired by empirical and unconscious reasoning, but this obscure and spontaneous march of the mind has been developed by the scientist into a clear and reasoned method which then proceeds more rapidly and consciously towards a set goal." [1]

Thus Claude Bernard, who was an incomparable experimentor, has given us very clear notions on the theory of inventions.

[1] Claude Bernard, *Introduction à la méthode expérimentale*, Paris, 1850, pp. 28, 33, 45, 54, 73.

II. The Unconscious in the Case of Experimentalists

1. *Claude Bernard and his researches on Sugar*

Claude Bernard gives us a brilliant example of the unforeseen discoveries which he mentioned. As the result of several experiments, he was brought to a conclusion exactly contrary to his theory.

He studied the phenomena of nutrition and noticed the important place occupied by sugar. He found it to be present in the intestinal mucous membranes, in the liver, in the sub-hepatic veins, in the right side of the heart, and in the lungs. On the other hand, sugar was wanting or at least rare in the left side of the heart and in the arteries. Hence Bernard concludes that sugar is absorbed by the intestinal mucous membranes, then transmitted to the liver and to the sub-hepatic veins to be carried to the heart and thence to the lungs, where it is burnt. Such was his opinion : it was the conclusion of his first conscious researches.

But one day an unexpected fact, altogether unforeseen, attracted his attention : The urine of diabetics contains a quantity of sugar greater than that found in the feculent or sweet foods which form part of their diet. Whence does this surplus come ? Evidently from another source than the intestinal canal which conducts away alimentary sugar coming from outside. Immediately the physiologist produced his hypothesis : the organism creates sugar somewhere.

The site of its production could be found by methodical tests. He gave doses of glucose along the whole length of the circulatory system, starting from the intestines. After its passage through the liver and through the sub-hepatic veins, the blood is richer in glucose than in the portal vein, at its entry into the liver. Without a doubt, " the excess can only come from the liver." The hypothesis was thus verified and made more precise.

However, in order to allow no room for criticism,

Claude Bernard tried a confirmatory experiment. " He fed a dog exclusively on meat for a greater or less time, a food the digestion of which could not give rise to glucose, and proved that the blood of the portal vein in front of the liver is absolutely devoid of glucose, while that of the sub-hepatic veins, after the liver, contains it in abundance : here the glucose comes entirely from the liver. The liver thus produces glucose incessantly which it pours into the blood : this is its glycogenic function.

The fact appears to be proved ; nevertheless, protests are uttered. Up till then it had been believed that only vegetables could produce immediate principles, and now it appeared that animals were producers of glucose. Thus his discovery not only contradicted Bernard's own original opinion, but it was entirely unexpected by the majority of physiologists.

This opposition suggested to Claude Bernard the decisive experiment which was to close the discussion. He showed that if a current of water is passed through the blood vessels of a liver detached from the body, a time comes when the liver has been completely washed out and no longer contains any trace of glucose. If now the liver be exposed to a temperature similar to that of the body, glucose is found in it in abundance after a few hours. This experiment makes it impossible to deny formation of sugar in the liver." [1]

If we analyze the five stages of this discovery from the psychological point of view, we find four conscious operations and a fifth partially unconscious.

(1) After studying the phenomena of nutrition, Bernard came to the conclusion that sugar, after being absorbed by the intestinal vessels and transmitted to the liver and to the sub-hepatic veins, is carried to the heart and then to the lungs, to be consumed there. Such was his erroneous opinion. It was the conscious preparation for his discovery.

[1] Van Tieghem, *Notice sur la vie et les travaux de Claude Bernard.*

(2) A fact struck him: the sugar of diabetics is greater than that corresponding to the food taken. The guiding idea immediately sprang into his mind : sugar is produced in the organism. Although preceding the experiments which were to prove it, this idea is a certain conclusion, but one logically anticipated. The conclusion is sudden ; but the latent reasoning which led to it contains partially unconscious elements, for subjective certainty precedes the experimental examination of the various possibilities which have to be taken into account.

(3) Three experiments follow : (a) that of dosing glucose along the whole length of the circulatory system. At the exit from the liver the quantity of sugar has increased : hence it comes from the liver. (b) The experiment of making glucose disappear before the passage of the blood to the liver, and then finding it reappear in the blood leaving the liver. (c) That of washing liver, and then placing it in a temperature about that of the body. In this case the liver alone could have been the creator of the glucose. These experiments, which were suggested by the hypothesis, represent three lines of reasoning in which all the propositions are clearly conscious. The relationship between them, by which one suggests the next, is perceived in full consciousness.

Thus the sole case of the unconscious which we can retain in this beautiful physiological discovery is that found in the sudden conception of the guiding idea, accompanied by complete subjective certainty. Thus in the case of Bernard, as in the case of so many others, conscious work preceded and followed the unconscious development.

2. Haüy and his Crystallography

The chance circumstances in which the Abbe Haüy was led to invent crystallography deserve notice. They were as follows :—

"One day, when examining some minerals at the house of one of his friends, he was fortunately clumsy enough to allow a beautiful cluster of prismatic crystals of calcspar to fall on the ground. One of the prisms broke in such a way as to show at the fracture faces which were no less smooth than those elsewhere, but presented the appearance of a new crystal altogether different in form from the prism. Haüy picked up this fragment and examined the faces with their inclinations and angles. To his great surprise, he discovered that they are the same in rhomboidal spar as in Iceland spar.

"He wished to be able to generalize : he broke his own little collection into pieces ; crystals lent by his friends were broken ; everywhere he found a structure which depended upon the same laws."

This observation, which was corroborated by further experiment, led him to formulate the laws of crystallography.

His previous studies, his more distant preparations for this discovery of a significant phenomenon had been logical and conscious.

He then made his interesting observation. Immediately he was ready to generalize, because he had seen the law behind the fact, because he had divined an infinity of other cases ruled by the same principle. His conclusion would be hasty if made by a logician demanding repeated and decisive proof, but it was not so for him. He suddenly sprang over the logical intermediates, as if forced by an unconscious necessity. It is in this haste that we find traces of unconscious work. Once again, we have found a phase of the unconsciousness succeeding conscious preparation, and followed by numerous conscious verifications.[1]

3. Louis Pasteur : Theory and Practice

Pasteur made numerous discoveries. As a result of them, he invented a general method of curing several

[1] Loridan, op. cit., p. 144.

diseases. It is this method which we are going to consider here.

In his case, conscious preparation was long and detailed. As a child he read a great deal. He was a good draughtsman and made portraits ; he had a taste for symmetry and a lively feeling for beauty. Further before studying biology he interested himself in crystals. Their regular configuration gave him a glimpse of the more general order of living beings ; crystallography and chemistry were to conduct him to the intensive analysis of the infinitely small units of life.

He was trained by Dumas at the Sorbonne, and "he was the disciple of the enthusiasm which this scientist inspired in him ".[1] In his case it was impossible to separate theory and practice. This is how he formulated his principles :—

"Without theory, practice is only routine given by custom. Theory alone can cause the spirit of invention to arise and develop. It is for you (his pupils), above all, not to share the opinion of those rigid minds which disdain everything in science which has no immediate application." [2]

On the other hand, he recommends conscious preparation. In a lecture given at Lille in 1856, he says : " In the field of observation, chance only favours minds which are prepared." He says more explicitly, in a work published in 1871 : " Discoveries, too, have their hidden and invisible germs which are productive or sterile to a degree determined by their preparation by genius, work, long striving, which are for them the source of life and fertility." [3]

This preparation is to be made in the first place by teaching, since it comprises a certain fund of general knowledge, which is the fertile source of the combinations

[1] Vallery-Radot, *La vie de Pasteur*, p. 25.

[2] *Documentation catholique*, No. 306, 24th Oct., 1925, p. 681.

[3] Pasteur, *Quelques réflexions sur la science en France*, Paris, 1871, p. 27.

of genius : " Scientists ought to be professors ; they are
the better teachers. Furthermore, when giving a course
of public lectures, they are obliged to include in their
scope various sciences which have points of contact."[1]

The way in which discoveries and inventions are born
is as follows :—

First, there must be no systematic spirit ; " the
systematic spirit is incapable of building anything up
in the order of physical and natural sciences."

" We force Nature to reveal her secrets by experiments
which are refined, well-reasoned, and followed up . . ."
That is why " laboratories are the reflections of life and
fecundity ".

Further, if there is such a thing as chance in invention,
it profits only the seeker : " In our day chance only
favours invention for minds which are prepared for
discoveries by patient study and persevering efforts.
Great practical innovations, great improvements in
industry and the arts have all come from the laboratories
of learned physicists, of highly trained chemists, of
observers and naturalists of genius. " These great
innovations," says Cuvier, " are nothing but easy
applications of truths of a superior order, of truths which
have not been sought for with this end in view, and
whose authors have only pursued them for their own
sake and have been urged on by the passion for
knowledge."[2]

Finally, Pasteur recognises that these fertile ideas are
often born of necessity : " Saltpetre is scarce ; it no
longer comes from India : Monge finds it in France and
makes gunpowder from it. The art of making steel is
created for the sake of the bayonet, the sword, the lance,
etc.—balloons will be developed to spy upon the enemy.
Numerous inventions were thus made during the French
Revolution, thanks to Monge, Carnot, Berthollet."[3]

---

[1] Op. cit., pp. 21, 22.
[2] Op. cit., p. 31.
[3] Op. cit., p. 39.

Regarded thus, these innovations are a triumph for reason : "Great discoveries introduce into the whole social system the philosophic or scientific spirit, that discerning spirit which submits everything to severe reasoning, condemns ignorance and dissipates prejudices and errors. They raise the intellectual and moral level. Through them, the divine idea itself is spread and exalted."

But the development of these precious germs must be assisted. Here Pasteur adopts the following thought of Claude Bernard : " New ideas and discoveries are like seeds ; it is not sufficient to give birth to them and to sow them ; they must be nourished and developed by scientific culture ; without it, they die or rather they emigrate, and then we see them prosper and fructify in the fertile soil which they have found far from the country which has given birth to them.

As an experimentor he proceeded in his discoveries by implacable logic. When at the *École normale supérieure* he one day left his laboratory very much moved, " seeking for someone to whom he could communicate the joy in his mind " : he had just separated the double para-tartrate of sodium and ammonium into two salts of opposite rotatory power for polarized light. It was his first discovery. One might suppose it to be a small matter, but one would be wrong. It was a revelation of a whole world of new things. From his close mathematical and physical studies there resulted his researches on crystallography, on hemihedry and on rotatory power, and these revealed to him the order which unites the great laws of nature. He found this order again in the arrangement of atoms, and he became one of the creators of stereochemistry. He found it again among the infinitely small living world and created microbiology.

He studied ferments, particularly the fermentation of beer, examined the technique of sterilizing cultures in order to perfect it, raised the temperature above 100° in order to kill microbes, and announced to the scientific world the use of the autoclave and the Pasteur oven for obtaining complete sterilization. Following the same order of ideas, he filtered microbes from the air by cotton wool, and thus endowed his successors with the culture tubes which are used to-day.

He then suspected that fermentation was a vital phenomenon, while Claude Bernard and Buchner had supposed it to be due to a soluble ferment. In order to prove this, he studied wines, beers, vinegar, pure yeasts and perfected yeasts.

Now, these yeasts might be able to explain the diseases of silk worms, so he proceeded to study the *pébrine* or silkworm disease. He was thus led to introduce the microscope.

He then passed from the diseases of animals to those of man, or rather, to those which are common to animals and man. He guessed the existence of microbes in anthrax and in chicken cholera, etc.

It was a chance which led him to the theory of immunization. One day an old and forgotten culture was being used for inoculating fowls. The fowl became ill but did not die : for they were immunized or vaccinated.

This was a ray of light. Pasteur set up this hypothesis, which was a hasty conclusion which had to be justified in the sequel : immunization by cultures of less and less virulence must be a law.

It was necessary to prove it. On the one hand, Jenner, without making any generalization, had assumed this law in its application to protection from smallpox. On the other hand, Pasteur's experiment on fowls afforded a second proof. He continued, feeling sure of the results, to multiply experiments.

He attacks anthrax, a very virulent disease. First, he is certain that a drop of blood infected with anthrax, when placed in nutritive bouillon at a temperature of 35°, develops the disease : he finds filaments enclosing spores. Pasteur sprinkles this bouillon on lucerne mixed with thistles, and allows sheep to eat it : the spines inoculate them with the disease, and they die a few hours afterwards of anthrax. The same results are obtained if cows are infected.

A surprise now occurs, which allows Pasteur to formulate the theory of immunization. The cows innoculated with anthrax do not always die ; further, they finally are able to resist the most active cultures. This is an indication. Pasteur submits a culture of bacilli to a temperature of 42°. No more toxin, no more spores : its very attenuated virulence should produce slight illness, and nothing more. And in fact, at Pouilly-le-Fort, near Melun, twenty-five sheep thus innoculated resist the injurious action of blood infected with anthrax, while twenty-five sheep which have not been vaccinated perish at the end of the third day.

If vaccination is operative against anthrax, is it capable of producing immunity to rabies ? Pasteur had a predecessor in this line of research. Bourrel, a veterinary surgeon, invented a method of protecting dogs against rabies. He filed the teeth of dogs to prevent their being able to break the skin. This was a mechanical procedure which suggested to Pasteur a more scientific method— vaccination against rabies.

First of all, where in the animal with rabies is the seat of the disease to be found ? Pasteur " collected facts in order to have ideas ". He experimented in turn on rabbits and dogs. He studied the slaver of mad dogs, then their nervous system, and arrived at this conclusion : rabies is not in the slaver alone, it is mainly in the nervous system.

Hence the remedy will have to do with the nervous system. The virus of rabies was cultivated from the spinal cord, and it is found that the ageing of this culture attenuated its virulence. After fourteen days dessication, the spinal marrow had lost its virulence altogether.

Now the period of incubation of rabies is a long one, as the facts prove. Hence it could be treated before its development. Pasteur experimented with perfect success on dogs which had been bitten ; he then experimented on man.

The way in which he healed the youths Meister and Jupiles in his laboratory at the Rue d'Ulm is well known. We may recall the stages of his method :—

(1) He removed the spinal marrow of rabietic rabbits.

(2) He dried it over calcium chloride.

(3) He arranged in a series marrows extracted after one day, two days, and so on up to fourteen days.

(4) He first injected the fourteen-day marrow, then that of the twelfth day, and so on, ending with that of the second day.

The theory of the result is as follows. The fourteen-day marrow produces a slight malaise in the patient, but at the same time renders him more resistent. He is thus able to take the twelve-day marrow, the ten-day, and so on. Finally he is inoculated with the very virulent product from the two-day marrow. But the previous inoculations have accustomed him to the virus and rendered him able to resist it at its full virulence. He is immunized.

With this we may close the history of Pasteur's discoveries. His work is a tissue of discoveries obtained by an admirable method, personal to himself, which was afterwards utilized by Chantemesse, Roux and Calmette. Pasteur's invention was this scientific procedure, and we may now seek to discover in its various phases whatever traces of the unconscious exist in it.

Pasteur's early history, a work of serene reason and serious criticism, was a long conscious preparation for scientific invention. He studied crystals, he followed Dumas' lectures, he studied deeply physics and mathematics, he founded stereochemistry, he began his experiments on yeast, etc.

He then observed two facts which precipitated the conclusions of his theory : (1) He saw that fowls do not succumb to inoculation by old cultures. (2) He noticed that cows do not always die of anthrax. Hence this hypothesis, a hasty generalization in relation to the experiment : Cultures of less and less virulence immunize the organism. Certain of the result, five years before the first cure of hydrophobia, he cried aloud in the laboratory, in the presence of his fellow workers at Rue d'Ulm :—

" Ah ! my friends, it is too beautiful ! . . . if my experiments are correct, there will be no more deaths from hydrophobia."

He experimented for five years. We come to the year 1885. The boy Meister, who had suffered fourteen bites from a mad dog, was brought to him. For eight days and nights without sleeping, almost without eating and drinking, Pasteur applied his treatment. Finally, after thirteen days, Meister was saved.[1]

The unconscious appears in this series of analogies which led Pasteur to pass from the study of yeast to that of pebrine, from pebrine to anthrax from anthrax to hydrophobia. In the mental syntheses which inspired the whole series of his experiments, Pasteur proceeded with assurance towards a goal which was glimpsed in the unconscious or subconscious penumbra. There was certainly evidence of the unconscious in the psychical work which made him so sure of the result. Nevertheless, it was simply the precipitation of a sudden conclusion : the unconscious logic, of which we have so often shown the necessity without exaggerating its range.

It is evident that, in Pasteur's case, conscious verification completed the latent work of the unconscious ; this is abundantly proved by what we have related of his discoveries. Nevertheless, we should note that it would be wrong to assign a precise place to logical confirmation in the magnificent series of his experimental demonstrations. In Pasteur's case, discoveries and inventions excite and follow one another like a series of rockets in the night. Every verification of a preconceived hypothesis is at the same time the preparation for a second invention, the leading idea of which is on

[1] Du Saussois, Pasteur, op. cit., pp. 35-9.

the point of bursting forth. Thus, in this powerful and well-ordered mind, there is an interpenetration of discoveries and inventions to such an extent that the interwoven preparations and verifications form a fabric in which the eye of the psychologist discerns shadows of the unconscious and high lights of logic, but which when seen from afar seems like a huge luminous structure.

4. *Darwin, the Inventor of Evolution*

In Pasteur's case, we have studied the invention of a rigorously exact scientific method. In Darwin's case, we have to examine an invention of another order ; a scientific theory sufficiently general to explain a great number of facts, but still hypothetical in certain respects, since its experimental proof remains incomplete. It is none the less a true invention ; it is a system with its bases and its laws ; it is a combination of principles from which science will, without doubt, draw certain conclusions in the future, just as the world of stars developed from the primitive nebula.

This great synthesis was not formed suddenly by a single crystallization ; it was a germ which developed little by little by the assimilation of numerous observations and successive experiments until it attained the proportions of a scientific system. The first idea of it came into Darwin's mind as follows. Darwin had seen in South America neighbouring species replacing one another from north to south, similar species in the islands off the coast and on the Continent, and finally, close relationship connecting toothless mammals and living rodents with extinct species of the same families.

Darwin felt himself able to draw from these observations the hypothetical conclusion, that species could descend from a common ancestor. This was the directing idea.

This idea was not absolutely new. Darwin knew this. He consulted his predecessors : Lamarck, who wrote his *Philosophie zoologique* from 1801 to 1809, and in 1815 his *Histoire naturelle des animaux sans vertèbres* ; Geoffroy-Saint-Hilaire, who, in 1795, suspected that " species were the descendants of a single type " ; Grant, who in 1826 in his *Memoire sur les spongilles* stated that " every species descends from other species and is improved by successive modification " ; Haldeman who, in 1843 and 1844, taught " the variability of species by accumulated modifications " ; finally H. Spencer, Huxley and Goethe, who believed that species could be improved by cultivation.

These views formed for Darwin a body of valuable previous work of which he had fully conscious knowledge. The intellectual tendency to believe in the transformation of species existed. His predecessors had spoken of improvements and modifications. He went further : he had the idea of a transformation by which one species could become another species. This was his personal invention, at the stage of an hypothesis.

It was necessary to verify it. To this end he studied plants and animals, circulated printed questionnaires, and accumulated notes and abstracts.

Incidentally, he made an observation which was particularly fertile in results. In order to propagate a species, man makes a choice. For him selection is the great factor in transformation. Thus, there arose in his mind the following idea, suggested by the foregoing observations : Might not this choice be general, might not selection be a law common to animals and plants, directing them in the transmission of life ?

His first hypothesis was made more definite ; species are transformed by *selection*.

At this moment, his attention was drawn to the book by Malthus on the principle of population. He read it for recreation and remarked the importance attached in it to the struggle for existence : " I had been well prepared by prolonged observation of animals and plants to appreciate the struggle for existence which is met with everywhere, and the idea struck me that in these circumstances, favourable variations would tend to be preserved, and other less privileged would be destroyed." [1]

Here was a new element which completed his hypothesis : Species are changed by selection as a result of the struggle for existence.

The whole of his work on the *Origin of Species by Natural Selection* is an account of numerous observations by which the author verified his hypothesis. The original character of the example which Darwin gives us is the following. His hypothesis is progressive ; it passes from an indefinite form to a more definite form by a slow process of unconscious evolution. We may summarize the decisive steps as follows :—

(1) After his voyage to South America, Darwin felt able to make the assumption that species might very well descend from a common ancestral form. This was a vague hypothesis, a simple possibility.

(2) After reading his predecessors and making personal observations, Darwin, fascinated by the idea of choice, made his thought more precise : transformations are brought about by selection.

(3) After reading Malthus and observing plants and animals over a long period, Darwin added the last feature to his hypothesis : transformations are accomplished by selection resulting from the struggle for existence.

Thus in the hypothesis itself there was clearly progress ; successive conclusions were elaborated in silent period, just as a rocket passes through the sky, leaving a faint track and producing luminous outbursts at intervals.

Thus in Darwin's case as in the case of so many others, the first observations and the last verifications were conscious. The slow modifications of this hypothesis was less so ; it expanded and extended by annexations which were unsuspected at their origin.

---

[1] See Charles Darwin's correspondence, with an autobiographical chapter, published by his son, Francis Darwin.

Summary and Conclusion

Inventions are preceded by a need or a desire, prepared for by intense conscious study, and followed by long processes of verification which are conscious.

(1) The part played by feeling is evident in the origin of invention: " Feeling always takes the initiative, it engenders the idea *a priori*," says Claude Bernard. Before discovering anything, Pasteur had a lively feeling for beauty, a taste for symmetry, and shared the noble enthusiasm of his master Dumas ; he recognized that fertile ideas are " daughters of necessity ". It was the desire for healing a part of humanity which accounted for his cries of joy five years before his method was verified. Finally, it was the desire to unite under one general law all the reflections suggested to him by his observations, that caused Darwin to invent his theory.

(2) A long conscious preparation preceded these discoveries of genius. Ten years of lectures and observations led Cuvier to his laws. In Grasset's case, the discoveries effected by the higher conscious psychism were only possible by means of the elements stored in the polygon, and we know that these elements are the residues of previous conscious activity. According to Claude Bernard, the *quid proprium* of the invention germinates in minds predisposed to it ; his discovery of the glycogenic function followed upon his long studies of the phenomena of nutrition. Haüy had made a long examination of crystals before he discovered their laws. Pasteur had studied deeply almost all sciences before inventing his theory of immunization. In the same way Darwin formulated his bold theory after long years of critical observation.

(3) The invention thus prepared for appears. What does it consist of ? Where is the unconscious element ? In Cuvier's case, it was a logical synthesis, and the unconscious is to be found in the invisible but real connections which had rendered possible the production

of his synthesis. For Hartmann and Schmidt, the unconscious is the instinctive phase which precedes and prepares the conscious phase in all intellectual work. Grasset regards the polygonal unconscious as ruminating and developing, while the higher psychism directs and produces the invention properly so called. In the case of Claude Bernard, there was in turn the invention of experiments and the discovery of laws, and the unconscious exists as well in the empirical instruction acquired, as in the preparation of an unexpected conclusion, which, one fine day, reveals the invention itself. In Pasteur's case, invention consists in every directing idea which comes to mark out the course of experimental reasoning, and there are fringes of the unconscious in the obscure process which results in these ideas bursting forth before the logical confirmation which they must receive from experiment. Finally, in Darwin's case, there was invention at each new step in the progress made in his hypothesis, invention in the elements which one by one were added to the first formula. There are also traces of the unconscious in the transition from one formula to another, that is to say, in the mysterious process which brings the scientist little by little towards his final system ; a certain degree of unconsciousness, since the first rough draft could not allow the final lines to be divined ; but a limited degree of unconsciousness, since Darwin, who was a careful and very critical observer, connected together very solidly the various elements which form his theory.

(4) The preceding analysis renders it unnecessary for us to insist on conscious verification. In order to effect it, Cuvier reconstructed the skeleton of every species bone by bone ; Grasset multiplied the functions of the higher psychism, of the centre O " it set moving, it directs, it revitalizes the polygon ". Claude Bernard, a true foreman of creation, invented phenomena and established by a crucial test that liver when warmed generates sugar. Haüy broke his collection of crystals

into pieces and thus founded crystallography. Finally Pasteur and Darwin did not tire of paying court to Nature by multiplying and varying experiments and observations and were happy to find that their hypothesis acquired, by being shown to be a general law, the glory of a rational system.

If we compare these results to those which have been obtained in the study of inventions produced in the domain of the physical sciences, we find that the unconscious plays a role which is perhaps more extended, but at any rate more varied. This difference is explained by the fact that the laws of biology are very complex and are discovered by observation followed by experiment. It is the observations in particular which suggest hypotheses formed little by little and slowly, by mysterious process of synthesis the logical steps of which are too disconnected to appear definitely in consciousness. The result is an unconscious which is not the less operative for being fragmentary; it provokes new observations, it generates, at distinct intervals, the various elements which, as we have seen in Pasteur's case and particularly in Darwin's, will form the final hypothesis.

Thus life, by bringing into science greater difficulty resulting from greater complexity, prolongs and multiplies in an inventive intelligence a period of unconscious incubation.

CHAPTER V

THE UNCONSCIOUS AND INVENTION IN THE MORAL SCIENCES

General procedure : Gustave Le Bon, Maine de Biran, Goethe, Souriau, Joly—The unconscious in the moral sciences properly so called : Aslan, Guyau—Invention in history : Seignobos—Invention in social science : Tarde—Invention in philosophy : Descartes, Nietzsche, A. Comte, Rignano and Goblot.

UNDER the term *moral sciences*, we understand in this book those sciences which seek for the laws of individual activity in its free manifestations. On their theoretical side, they teach us human affairs as they are. In this group is included psychology, history, philology, and sociology. In their practical or normative form, they determine the ideal laws to which human liberty conforms ; these are logic, morality properly so called, æsthetics, practical politics, political economy, and jurisprudence in their respective parts. The method of the first class is before all the inductive, that is to say, it is based upon observation. The method of the second is principally deductive ; it indicates the rules to be followed in order to reach a given ideal. Nevertheless, this distinction has certainly been exaggerated. Induction and deduction, being general methods, are necessary to all moral sciences ; for theoretical sciences need deduction to deduce the practical consequences of established laws ; on the other hand, the practical sciences make use of induction in order to learn the nature of man, to which they are to trace logical rules or moral standards. These

151

standards, which are very different from the laws of physics and chemistry, are not inevitable ; they apply to facts which are difficult to foresee, and are not simply indicative ; they are the rules of an obligatory ideal. It follows that inventions in this domain must make use of two factors apparently opposed to one another ; determinism, which is inherent in all science, and human liberty, which is the postulate of all moral life. By reason of this conflict, inductions will be long, and generalization hazardous and difficult. In the course of the long process of reasoning which leads to an invention, many unperceived causes will modify the premises. We thus see, *a priori* in what zone the unconscious, which inspires discoveries relating to these sciences, must be situated. This being so, we will proceed to examine the general methods followed in discoveries of this nature, and then see in what way these methods vary in moral science properly so called, in history, in sociology and in philosophy.

I.   The GENERAL PROCEDURE IN MORAL INVENTION

1.   *Gustave Le Bon and the Theory of Residues*

The first problem is the existence of invention in general and of any particular invention. Gustave Le Bon gives us a plausible explanation :—

" Since the bonds connecting things are innumerable, our observations and explanations of phenomena can never be complete. There thus remains in every explanation, *residues*, the origin of which will be sought for by a more advanced science. The interpretation of these residues always leads to some discovery." [1]

According to this author, therefore, the first cause

---

[1] Le Bon, *La vie des vérités*, op. cit., p. 240.

of scientific research is a statement of fact. A part of the vast field of knowledge has been cleared, that is to say explained or elucidated ; but another part remains unexplored, certain points of a theory remain obscure, the demonstration is incomplete. The need for discoveries or inventions thus becomes an appeal for further explanation.

Fundamentally, this is a *desire* for deeper knowledge, and on this point Maine de Biran carries further the views of Gustave Le Bon.

2. *Maine de Biran : Feeling at the Origin of New Ideas.*

He makes first of all this categorical declaration : " Only a fixed feeling can bring fixed ideas ".

There follows a confession, which is the consequence of the preceding :—

" In youth, all our ideas are in agreement with the feelings which excite them and have a vivacity, a particular attraction, which animates our inward life . . . I was much happier of old in solitude, etc." (A personal example.)

We thus have, according to Biran, feeling at the base of the idea. The transition from one to the other must take place when the feeling has acquired a certain coefficient of intensity :—

" There are times, days, moments, when the feeling principle seems to pierce through the clouds which obscure it. These are the flashes of light which suddenly illuminate my mind, but the darkness only appears deeper afterwards."[1]

Biran's confidences thus lead us to Poincaré's sudden illuminations. Moreover, an unconscious process causes us to pass from the feeling to the idea.

[2] Maine de Biran, *Sa vie et ses pensées*, by E. Naville, p. 153, Paris, 1857. *Année*, 1811, p. 145 ; *Année*, 1815.

The intermediary of this passage is the creative imagination applied to knowledge of the moral order. But in order to fertilize it, it must be furnished and enriched by the acquisitions from frequent meditative reading.

3. *Relative Fields of Consciousness and the Unconscious according to Goethe, Souriau, and Joly*

In general, we may thus distinguish the zones of the consciousness and the unconscious in inventions relating to moral science in the following manner :—

" Desire appears first . . . Our desires, says Goethe, are the presentiment of faculties in ourselves, the precursors of things which we are capable of executing."

As a result of reading, or of intellectual communion of some kind with others, certain ideas penetrate into the mind. The sum total of these ideas, and their connection with one another—that is to say the connection of the last one with the preceding—are the conscious phenomena, says P. Souriau. We take them into account.

But what is unconscious, adds the same writer, is the bond which links present ideas to the idea of a future reaction. Consequently, no invention can be intentional. The images constructed by the imagination are developed by annexations, the origin of which is unsuspected. The essential idea constituting the invention supervenes ; in a sense it is without precedent among preceding ideas ; it is thus original, or at least, appears to be so. Its kinship with antecedent conceptions, is, however, undeniable. But the point of attachment remains unperceived. We thus see, in the constructive work of the imagination, necessary logical connections, but unconscious ones.

Let us examine in detail, in the various forms of the moral sciences, the extent of these obscure zones.

II. THE UNCONSCIOUS IN MORAL SCIENCE PROPERLY SO CALLED

1. *Inventions in morals according to Aslan and Guyau*

As an example of an invention, in the sense of the elaboration of a theoretical system of morals, we may examine the ideas of G. Aslan.[1]

First we have the occasion of these inventions. Moral invention takes place after moral crises, and these crises are useful: "They are the promisers of renewal, of rejuvenation," says Auguste Comte. "The innovators in the field of morals are neither pure negators, nor the discouraged who take refuge in scepticism. They seek a more living and a purer ideal."

Now the doctrine of this author in morals is rationalism: "Belief can only derive its authority from its agreement with a rational principle, in the same way that the thought of the scientist passes beyond the fact of experience in order to formulate a scientific law. Consequently, in the invention of a system of morals, we need both the facts of experience to determine the good and a "restrictive" rational interpretation to define the limits of the moral intuition which is the result of experience.

Aslan, following in this point Guyau's principles, thus arrives at the reduction of invention in morals to a syllogism with the following three propositions:—

Major : The human will seeks the good in general.

Minor : The facts of experience give us the determination of this good.

Conclusion : The will thus follows a moral rule drawn from experience and solely within the limits of its agreement with a rational principle.

It is not a matter for us to discuss the logical value of this syllogism in this place, since we are dealing with

[1] Aslan (G.), *Expérience et invention en morale*, Paris, 1908, pp. 2, 22, 142.

psychology. We may only note the place of experimental facts in the elaboration of this system. There is an intuition, and then a deduction based upon the intuition. And because experience must be extended, intuition must be manifold. We immediately see that, thanks to these intuitions, the idea of the conclusion will be anticipated before the proof is finished. We thus return to a phase of semi-consciousness which must be judged necessary to explain the precipitate conclusion of the syllogism.

2. *Invention in Morals according to Le Bon*

In more general terms than Aslan, Le Bon builds up the whole of individual morals by underlining the modifications produced in the character by the passage from the rules of conduct imposed from without, to moral laws unconsciously formed by the repetition of acts.

" By means of the unconscious, he writes, we come to do what we ought to do . . . The act which is repeated is automatized by the unconscious, and is accomplished without effort. This is how the soldier marches in step without thinking about it, and the pianist, in order to cause a certain note to be sounded, touches, without reflection, a part of the piano producing this note . . . Individual morality is first imposed, and then passes into the unconscious by education. The great progress of social life would result from this substitution of an unconscious morality accepted without effort for a conscious morality which could only be enforced by severe punishment." [1]

We may leave it to the moralist to observe the fragility of a moral edifice founded on unconscious automatism, and simply retain these two statements :—

(1) In a first, conscious stage, vigorous punishment has inculcated into individuals the notions of good and evil.

[1] Le Bon, op. cit., pp. 178–9.

(2) In an unconscious stage, as the result of habit, the great principles of morality have been engraven on the human soul. They are thus imposed as standards which must be followed without our knowing the true motives at the base of their obligatory character.

In this case, there was doubtless a conscious preparation. People must have been conscious of the strokes of the whip received by way of moral preparation. But no light of inspiration can have shone in the eyes of the moral slave. Finally, no conscious verification is possible since we pass insensibly from the consciousness to the unconscious.

III. THE UNCONSCIOUS IN HISTORICAL INVENTION

Seignobos and the Synthetic construction of the image representing the Historical fact

With great precision, Seignobos analyses the various phases of the work of historical reconstitution.

There are a number of conscious operations, such as relate to research, scrutiny, criticism, and reasoned utilization of documents. The historian who is worthy of the name, consults bibliographies, seeks, in his criticisms of origins, the sources from which authors have drawn ; establishes, in his textual criticism, the concordance between the actual text and the primitive text, and examines what the author has said, whether he believes what he said, and whether he was justified in believing it.

At this moment, a partially unconscious operation is accomplished : " A phrase of a document has been read. An image is formed in our mind by a spontaneous operation over which we have no control. This is an analogy which is still superficial, an image which is perhaps crude and somewhat erroneous. The work of the historian consists in gradually rectifying our images

UNCONSCIOUS IN THE SCIENCES

by replacing one by one false characters by true characters." [1]

But this progressive rectification of the sketch-image, is, it may seem, a conscious labour. The only place which can be assigned to the unconscious is thus the formation of the primitive image, a kind of informal draft which is susceptible of both correction and development. This draft is the analogue of the hypothesis in physical science. Being traced without our knowledge by the imagination, it is less a creation properly so called than a fragmentary reconstruction of historical reality. The information derived from the sources consulted, the reflections suggested by the documents, have furnished the imagination with the material which it uses. Now a number of stones is not a wall without their being arranged, and joined to neighbouring stones by mortar. Thus a series of historical facts recalled to mind, do not form a synthesis unless the imagination cement together these stones placed side by side, by a mysterious cement, which is a true creation of the mind and explains the difference seen between two accounts of the same historical event. In this work of reconstructing the past, therefore, there is certainly creation, and hence invention. Hence, from the psychological point of view, the unconscious which presided at its elaboration, is either the imaginative unconscious or the rational unconscious found in all mental synthesis.

IV.   THE UNCONSCIOUS IN INVENTION IN THE SOCIAL SCIENCES

Tarde, Theorist and Practician of Invention

Tarde has given us an original theory of invention in order to make us understand his own personal invention, that of the laws of imitation.

---

[1] Seignobos, *Introduction aux études historiques*, Paris, 1910, pp. 30–7. 63, 192, 193.

He connects very ingeniously the explanation of discoveries and inventions with the theory of the interference of light. He regards the psychological interplay of a desire or a belief, or of two currents of imitation, or of a current of imitation or of an external perception, as a case of interference producing either an intensification or a dimunition and in either case a new entity, and consequently an invention.

" All inventions and discoveries being made up of elements of antecedent imitations, it follows that there is a general tree of these successful initiatives . . . Every invention which comes into being is a possibility realised among a thousand different possibilities." Why this one rather than that ? Because it responds to a need or satisfies a desire.   Tarde shows the necessity of this :—

" Inventions and discoveries which appear successively and are seized upon and made public by imitation, do not follow one another by chance ; a rational connection exists between them."   Now this connection is not necessarily thought of ; the scientist or inventor follows it in spite of himself.   There is thus an unconscious logical element in this series.

Nevertheless, although he is inspired by his environment, the inventor is not Society, but the individual : " The laws of invention belong exclusively to individual logic : The laws of imitation to social logic."

What is invention ?   " A mental encounter of knowledge already old and usually transmitted from others ; it is the interference of two thoughts, one of which modifies, attenuates, or reinforces the other ; in short it is the fertile interference of repetitions."

Understood thus, " inventions respond to a need for logical unification . . . discoveries are a gain in certitude, inventions a gain in confidence and security."

Tarde regards invention as a prolongation of imitation. " Now imitation may be voluntary, conscious or unconscious . . .

In the case of the individual, which ended by being an habitual unconscious, began by being a voluntary and conscious act. Many imitations are unconscious and involuntary from their origin."[1]

But invention goes beyond imitations as a building rises above its foundations. " What is invented is always an idea or a wish, a judgement or a design in which a certain element of belief or desire is expressed . . . "

In particular, " all social development is an increase in organization obtained by a relative diminution in action."

Progress is thus possible by social invention. " Progress is a kind of collective meditation without its own brain, but made possible by the solidarity of the many brains of inventors and scientists who exchange their successive discoveries."[2]

Now " social progress, like individual progress, takes place in two ways : Substitution and accumulation. There are discoveries and inventions which are only substitutable, others which are accumulatable. Hence logical battles and logical unions ".

In this combat as well as this union of thought, shadow will alternate with light ; there will be unforeseen events : " However, numerous may be the diverse varieties of things which repeat, if we imagine that the foci of these repetitive radiations—in other words, inventions—are regularly distributed, there encounters can be forseen. If, on the contrary, we admit that the primitive foci are irregularly dispersed, the secondary foci will also have an unordered arrangement, and there irregularity will be the greater, the greater that of the primitive foci."

Anyone can see the unconscious element in this inventive work. The dispersion of the foci will be the general case, the irregular dispersion the most frequent.

---

[1] Tarde, *Les lois de l'imitation*, pp. 160, 163.
[2] Op. cit., p. 161.

Thus, absence of prevision and unconsciousness, will frequently be necessary.

Tarde enlarges still further the field of invention. " Invention is not a simply category of work. It is the primary cause . . . of all riches, of all needs, and of a desire, of which riches are only the object. There is thus only a single true agent of production, invention, and three subordinate factors : Work, capital, and nature." [1]

We thus find ourselves led by this author to see traces of unconsciousness in all forms of human activity in the search for riches.

But Tarde is not content to be a theorist of invention. He himself experienced it, and this is how he was led to his discovery of the laws of imitation.

First of all, he sought for a doctrine in the opposite sense concerning universal difference, and the necessity, in the case of any reality, of differing from others.

But a fact appeared : He found likenesses and these likenesses embarrassed him. In order to justify his first theory, he considered these likenesses as the minima of difference.

However, their great number made him uneasy. Thereupon came the decisive fact which obliged him to change his hypothesis. One morning, in 1872, he was botanizing on a hill dominating the Valley of the Dordogne, in the neighbourhood of Laroque—Gajac, and his impressions were as follows :—

" I was struck with the likenesses which I found between the various categories of plants which I had just reviewed . . . I saw clearly that I had my finger on ideas of a fertility altogether different from that of the ideas which had hitherto been my guide ; nevertheless I did not immediately renounce them, but took the line of forgetting them for a time in order to give myself up entirely to the new point of view. After a few hours of walking and reflection, with several stops, I sat down

---

[1] Cf. Tarde, *Logique sociale*, quoted by Gide : *Principes d'économie politique*, pp. 110–12.

M

at the foot of a tree in order to make some notes in pencil, and made the first sketch of what afterwards became the first chapter of my *Laws of Imitation*, entitled 'Universal Repetitions'.

An encounter took place in my mind which is easily explained by my reading and reflections of the preceding days." [1]

Altogether we find in Tarde's case a magnificent example of association by contrast : There was produced the " reaction of a number of ideas formed in parallel to rival ideas ".

He had previously read the theory of physical waves. He said to himself by analogy : " Man in biology, plays the part of a complex wave which can be resolved into more simple living waves." He thought of the law of Malthus, generalized by Darwin : Every species tends towards indefinite progression through generalization—a law similar to that of light, of sound, of radiant heat. As a result of this reflection, " a day came when his ideas were co-ordinated into a general system together with the elements which escaped the first dominating ideas."

It is interesting to note that in this case the unconscious brought the erring seeker after truth back to the right path.

V. The Unconscious and Invention in the Philosophical Sciences

1. *Descartes and the Principle of his Psychology*

Descartes gives us the most typical example of the role of feeling and the unconscious in the elaboration of a new philosophy on a psychological basis.

His father's ancestors were doctors. He himself was fond of medicine ; his health was delicate. He studied

---

[1] Paulhan, *Psychologie de l'invention*, Paris, 1901, p. 20.

philosophy with passion, particularly St. Thomas Aquinas. He read *l'Art* of Lulle, and experienced the desire to find a general method applicable to all sciences. Experience had already shown him the superior value of sciences based upon certainty and evidence. In order to obtain good advice, he did not go to the theorists, he went to the army and made the acquaintance in 1618 of the physicist and mathematician Isaac Beeckman, who incited him to take up research : " I was asleep," Descartes wrote to him, " and you awakened me." After having been " in love with poetry, and fascinated by eloquence " he rose above these mental gifts which are not the fruits of study, and devoted himself by preference to mathematics. " On account of the evidence of reason," he revered theology but did not dare to submit revealed truth beyond our intelligence to his own weak reasoning powers, and was astonished to meet so much diversity in the opinions of philosophy. Since other sciences base their principles upon the latter, he concluded that it is impossible to " build anything solid on such insecure foundation ". Doubt descended upon him : Descartes doubted everything, the sensible world, since the senses deceive us, mathematics, since certain people have made mistakes in it ; he even imagines a God who deceives him, he doubts even himself, and doubts his own doubt, and stops at his doubt.

He was at this point on the 10th November, 1619, at Neubourg, near Ulm, " shut up the whole day in his chamber, without any cares or passions to trouble him, when he had a mystical crisis represented by three dreams, the little known details of which have been published by M. G. Maillet and M. J. Chevalier.[1]

This is the phase of unconsciousness which precedes the inventions.

His brain caught fire ; he fell into a state of enthusiasm.

[1] G. Maillet, " Une crise mystique chez Descartes," in *Revue de métaphysique*, July, 1916, p. 611. Chevalier (J.), *Descartes*, Paris, 1920, pp. 41–6.

On going to bed, still with this exaltation, he found that day the basis for the "admirable science".

First dream : He was driven in spite of himself towards a church. Then he was turned back. On awaking he felt a feeling of grief. In order to get rid of it, he prayed to God.

Second dream : He went to sleep again, heard thunder and seized with fear he saw flashes of fire. On awakening, he interpreted his dream : The fear was the remorse of his conscience ; the thunder was the " Spirit of Truth ", about to possess him.

Third dream : He saw a dictionary and the *Corpus Poetarum*. He found in these two books all human sciences manifested by the Spirit of Truth. He thought that poets, thanks to imagination and divine enthusiasm, find more intelligent maxims than those of philosophers. On the next day, he prays to God to enlighten him, and vows to make a pilgrimage to Lorette.

The sense of these three dreams, according to his own interpretation, was as follows :—

(1) This " admirable science ", the revealed principle of all science, must be sought in ourselves ; it is " like fire in flint ".

(2) It must be sought there, not by the reason of the philosophers " represented by the dictionary ", but by the inspiration of the poets (symbolized by the *Corpus Poetarum*), that is to say, by intuition, which develops these germs by making use of natural correlation between sensible things and spiritual things.

(3) The truth of this knowledge is guaranteed to us by the Spirit of Truth, that is to say, by God, who puts us on our guard against the illusions of the evil spirit and assures our reason of its value for science and wisdom.[1]

If we translate these apocalyptic declarations of Descartes into philosophical language, the result is as follows. Previous meditation has led the philosopher to doubt and revoke successively his previous beliefs.

[1] Chevalier, op. cit., pp. 44–6.

At the last, this question arises : Could God deceive him ? These ideas ferment in his mind which has become a laboratory of possible reaction. They meet there with religious ideas, hence this striving towards the church in the first dream, the fear and remorse of conscience in the second dream. There is also a conflict between pure reason and feeling. The latter triumphs : No, God could not deceive him, otherwise he would cease to be God.

It was thus with his heart of a Christian that he divined, by an intuition analogous to that of the poet, this great truth. *Intuition* as a method, *divine veracity* (Spirit of Truth) as guaranteed : Such were the consequences of the elaboration and conflicts of ideas effected during the three dreams. On awakening, suddenly, in the light of absolute evidence, Descartes grasps the necessity for intuition and divine veracity. Thus the three dreams were three distinct phases of unconscious ferment. And the three awakenings, analogous to the flashes in which Poincaré saw his discoveries, correspond with these three principles of his new philosophy : (1) We must start from the ego, by the reflective method, in order to found philosophy ; (2) The initial certainty is not obtained by reasoning, but is a truth of intuition ; the *cogito ergo sum* is thus equivalent to *cogito et sum cogitans* ; that is to say, I think and I am a thinking being : the expression of an intuitive truth, not the conclusion of a process of reasoning ; (3) *Divine veracity* is the necessary guarantee of knowledge. Absolutely, as in the case of mathematics, these three truths appear like three shining points ; they leave no room for any doubt. They constitute the invention properly so called following upon the unconscious incubation of the dream.

It is unnecessary to add that this mysterious work is followed by conscious operation. From the thinking ego, Descartes passes to the body distinct from the soul since he conceives himself as existing without thought being present ; he passes to the existence of God since he has within him the ideas of perfection and infinity, which cannot come either from nothing, or from himself, or from the external world, and hence must come from God. We thus find in this great mind, a mind so philosophical, that it seems with its love of truth to embrace the philosophy of all time, the influence of feeling and unconscious urges upon the rational orientation of a marvellous system of philosophy.

2. *Nietzsche and his Idea of Reincarnation*

Another thinker, Nietzsche, tells us in a much more obscure style how the idea of reincarnation came to him. This is what he writes in *Ecce Homo*.

" Suddenly, with a certainty and clarity which are indescribable, something becomes visible and spreads out, something which shakes us to the depth of our being and moves us. We listen, we do not speak ; we take, we do not ask who is giving ; like a flash a thought shines out, with necessity in its form, without hesitation ; it is an ecstasy, the excessive tension of which sometimes dissolves into a torrent of tears, while our steps, without our wishing it, sometimes hasten, sometimes slow down . . . One is completely beside oneself . . . All this is involuntary, like a storm of feelings of liberty, of power, of divinity . . ."

3. *Comte. The Inventor of the Religion of Humanity*

The career of Comte is interesting in view of the effect on his philosophy of his relationshlp with Clotilde de Vaux. This, as is well known, caused him to develop his religion of Humanity, in which the social elements were united by sympathy.

4. *Rigano and Goblot. The Unconscious in Invention and Logic*

The first of these philosophers, whose original conception of the nature of reasoning we shall discuss later, attempted to discover the nature of this logical operation ; he divided complex phenomena into their elementary simple elements " As long as I did not succeed in effecting this decomposition," he writes, " the complex psychical phenomenon remained for me an enigma . . . Finally, one fine day, at a moment when I least thought about the matter, I saw suddenly and clearly what I had been seeking in torment for a long time, that is to say, what appeared to be the true mechanism of reasoning, as it results from the combined play of the various activities of the mind." [1]

Goblot showed, in his *Essay on the Classification of the Sciences* that the syllogism does not take account of mathematical reasoning. He read this phrase of Duhamel's in his *Method of the Sciences of Reasoning* : " It is the art of directing the syllogism which makes the whole fertility of mathematics." He thus seeks to find what this art is, and this is the result : " It was at the end of ten years of research that the solution suddenly came into my mind, one morning in February, 1906, and it is an idea so simple that I cannot explain why I should have taken ten years to discover it : *deduction is construction*. We only demonstrate hypothetical judgments. We demonstrate that one thing is the consequence of another. For that purpose, we construct the consequence with the hypothesis." [2]

VI. SUMMARY AND CONCLUSION

As regards conscious preparation, it is long and varied all the philosophers we have considered illustrate this fact.

At the basis of all these researches, we find a lively desire.

[1] Rignano (Eugenio), *Psychologie du raisonnement*, Paris, 1920, Preface, p. viii.
[2] Goblot, *Le systeme des sciences*, pp. 50–1.

The constructive work of the imagination is considerable. This faculty, says Lenoble, conceives the end and the means ; it creates a new ideal to be attained, hastens the advent of truth by hypothesis, forms by analogy the sketch of an historic fact in an image which is gradually rectified.

CHAPTER VI

THE UNCONSCIOUS AND TECHNICAL INVENTION

The general character of technical invention—The invention of printing : the three successive suggestions—The invention of prime movers : Watt and the condenser, Stephenson and the locomotive—The Jacquard loom—Boring machines—Summary and conclusion.

TECHNOLOGY is the general study of the industrial arts, while technique is used to denote the various processes which are followed out in a special trade. The first is more theoretical ; the second is above all things practical. Having made this distinction, we shall henceforth ignore it. For whether theoretical or practical, each of these two sciences· is a rich source of invention, which usually takes the form of a machine.

I. THE GENERAL CHARACTER OF TECHNICAL INVENTIONS

(a) They require the active assistance of creative imagination

As we have said, the inventions in question most often take the form of machines. Now a machine is a complicated apparatus. It works by the interaction of a large number of parts, and this co-ordination of parts must be foreseen before it can be realized by the imagination. But the imagination does not create from nothing ; it associates in a new manner materials furnished by experience. Nevertheless, the more we know of various combinations, the better our chance of discovering new ones. Here we see the useful part played by the memory. By its revision of ideas and forms, it facilitates fortunate encounters and thus ensures inventive fertility.

(b) They are numerous and frequent as human desires themselves

A second character of these inventions is their frequency and variety. They cover the whole gamut of the desires and needs of humanity.

(c) Inventions are frequently a collective product

In the third place, we must agree with R. H. Thurston that great inventions and discoveries are seldom or never the work of a single man. Every great invention is in reality either a combination of several other secondary inventions, or the last result of a long continuous progress. It does not appear by sudden creation ; it grows little by little like the trees of the forest. It thus very often comes about that the same invention appears at the same time in different countries, having been made simultaneously by several people. Very frequently also, an important invention enters the world before the latter is ready to receive it, and the unfortunate inventor learns by his failure that it is not less disastrous to be ahead of one's time than to be behind it. For an invention to succeed, it is not merely necessary that it should fill a need, but also that humanity should be sufficiently advanced to appreciate it, to demand it, and to immediately make use of it.[1]

In this collaboration of inventors of genius, which we have seen in other sciences, but which is still more necessary in technology, we shall see, in spite of the discontinuity of the various attempts which have led to the final machine, how inventors inherit from their predecessors, are conscious of their own work, sometimes unconscious of the elements borrowed, and almost always unconscious of the mysterious logical process which connects together either their own successive personal inventions, or their own final inventions with those of their contemporaries.

[1] R. H. Thurston, *A History of the Steam Engine*, London, 1872, vol. i, pp. 2 and 3.

We may begin with Gutenberg, and the invention of printing.

II. INVENTION OF AN ESSENTIALLY INTELLECTUAL ART : PRINTING

The history of the discovery of this marvellous art is known to us by the letters written from the shores of the Rhine towards the middle of the fifteenth century by Gutenberg to Frère Cordelier.[1]

We quote in full the essential passages, adhering scrupulously to their strange form, their repetition, and their tone, at once simple and passionate. The defects in composition admirably exhibit the state of mind of the inventor tortured at each instant by the impatience of his desire to succeed.

(a) *At the origin, an ardent desire, a fixed idea : to simplify the laborious work of copyists*

We follow him in the various stages of his attempts and in the progress of his discovery.

First of all, he is burning to succeed. " For a month my head has been working ; a Minerva, fully armed, must issue from my brain . . . I wish to write by a single application of my hand, by a single movement of my fingers, in a single instant, and by a single effort of my thought, everything that can be put on to a large sheet of paper, lines, words and letters, by the labour of the most diligent class for a whole day, nay for several days." [2]

(b) *First suggestion of the means : Playing cards and pictures of the Saints*

" You have seen, as I have, playing cards and the pictures of Saints . . . these cards and pictures are engraved on small pieces of wood, and below the pictures

---

[1] *Histoire de l'invention de l'imprimerie par les monuments*, Paris, 1840.
[2] First letter.

there are words and entire lines also engraved . . . A thick ink is applied to the engraving ; and upon this a leaf of paper, slightly damp, is placed ; then this wood, this ink, this paper, is rubbed and rubbed until the back of the paper is polished. This paper is then taken off and you see on it the picture just as if the design had been traced upon it, and the words as if they had been written ; the ink applied to the engraving has become attached to the paper attracted by its softness and by its moisture

" . . . By multiplying these engraved pieces of woods, hundreds and thousands of copies are obtained by repeating the same operation.

" Well, what has been done for a few words, for a few lines, I must succeed in doing for large pages of writing, for large leaves covered entirely on both sides, for whole books, for the first of all books, the Bible . . .

" How ? It is useless to think of engraving on pieces of wood the whole thirteen hundred pages or of obtaining prints by rubbing, for one could not print the back of a page already charged wth ink on one side excepting at the expense of this first side, the writing on which would be rubbed out . . .

" What am I to do ? I do not know : but I know what I want to do : I wish to manifold the Bible, I wish to have the copies ready for the pilgrimage to Aix-la Chapelle . . ." [1]

The obsession of the desire to realize a work useful to religion reappears for the second time.

(c) *Second suggestion of the means :   the manufacture of coins*

" Every coin begins with a punch. The punch is a little rod of steel, one end of which is engrav?d with the shape of one letter, several letters, all the signs which are seen in relief on a coin. The punch is moist?ned and driven into a piece of steel, which becomes a hollow or

[1] First letter.

stamp. It is into these coin stamps, moistened in their turn, that are placed the little discs of gold, to be converted into coins, by a powerful blow." [1]

(d) Third suggestion of the means : The Press and the Seal

The idea of the punch had already called up the idea of pressure, for the punch is driven into the steel. Two recollections, that of the wine-press, and that of the seal complete the notion, when that of possible repetition is added.

" I took part in the wine harvest. I watched the wine flowing, and going back from the effect to the cause, I studied the power of this press which nothing can resist." Now this pressure might be exercised by means of lead. A simple substitution which is a ray of light, for the pressure exercised by the lead would leave a trace on paper. The inventor cried in triumph :—

" To work then ! God has revealed to me the secret that I demanded of him . . . I have had a large quantity of lead brought to my house, and that is the pen with which I will write."

It was then that the idea of necessary repetition was born : might not this leaden pen act in the same way as the seal used by the monks to sign their documents ? Evidently, and Gutenberg goes on :—

" When you apply to the vellum or paper the seal of your community, everything has been said, everything is done, everything is there. Do you not see that you can repeat as many times as necessary the seal covered with signs and characters ? "

Here we have then, to sum up the procedure to be employed : " One must strike, cast, make a form like the seal of your community, a mould such as that used for casting your pewter cups, letters in relief like those on your coins, and the punch for producing them like

---

[1] Second letter, p. 2.

your foot when it multiplies its print. There is the
Bible ! " [1]

The essentials of the invention were found. What
followed were the practical details of its realization.
First of all, Gutenberg rejected cursive and round-
writing : He chooses the form of his letters as follows :—

" I kept to a good letter of solid form, compact,
square, well-set ; I did not choose it, it came to me
prepared for my work by Providence. I have chosen
the large letter of the Missal."

Then he describes the making of the characters :
" First, the relief in steel, the punch carrying at its
extremity the engraved letter. Then the mould obtained
by driving the punch into copper : It is the mother of
the letters, the matrix ; then comes the mould in two
parts which interlock . . . "

Finally, movable letters are possible : " The metal
is thrown quickly down from above, while the shock
given to the moulds drives the melted metal into the
hollow of the matrix . . . You open the mould and
take out a small model in lead of the steel punch, a
little piece carrying at one end a delicate relief, at the
other end the rough fin, which has to be cut off. So we
have the letters, sisters like to one another, and like
the original punch."

Having obtained his letters, all that remains to be
done is to arrange them, an easy operation since they
are movable.

" The letters are movable, The mobility of the letters,
says the inventor, is the true treasure which I have been
searching for along unknown roads. With these letters
and with the blanks which give separation, I compose
words." [2]

These quotations are sufficient. They indicate clearly
the mental phenomena which, in Gutenberg's case,
preceded, accompanied and followed realization. We
may summarize them as follows :—

[1] Fifth letter.   [2] Eighth and ninth letters.

(e) Discussion

(1) First an intense desire presided over the researches, this desire being religious. Gutenberg wished to contribute to the diffusion of the Bible, the first of all books ; he wished to contribute to the success of the Pilgrimage to Aix-la-Chappelle.

(2) The successive inventions are three in number : the apparatus had to produce a picture, an image ; the apparatus had to be a press, a seal, the same way as the punch produces the coin. These three inventions are suggested by analogy : The cards and the pictures caused him to think of the form of a letter. The wine-press and the community seal caused him to think of pressure with lead, the coin and the punch which produces it awaken the idea of a similar punch : A triple analogy, the source of three partial inventions which complete one another.

(3) The unconscious which is present in all analogies, is therefore present in this three-fold conception of the apparatus ; we have as it were a movement of the mind in three distinct leaps, each of which renders possible the one following ; there is a triple movement of approach to the truth, each step resulting from the speed acquired during the one preceding.

(4) The ray of light on which the invention is founded, is revealed chiefly at two moments ; at the moment of the substitution of lead for the material in the wine-press, since from thenceforth printing is possible ; at the moment of the realization of multiple and mobile letters, since their mobility allows them to be arranged. Gutenberg confesses it. The secret revealed by God, was that of producing an imprint by means of lead (the ray of light) ; the mobility of letters, was the treasure sought for by unknown roads (the second ray of light).

(5) The small details of the operation are nothing more than the extension of the principal discovery ;

a conscious labour, just as the work of reflection suggested by each of the partial inventions had been conscious.

III.   THE INVENTION OF MACHINES RELATING TO TRANSPORT

1.   *The Steam Engine : Watt and his condenser*

The Englishman Watt, born in 1736, gives us a curious example of inventive work prepared over a long period and suddenly crowned by the discovery sought for. The whole of his youth was an initiation into the realities which were to make his fame. At six years of age, says Arago, he was already solving geometrical problems, experimenting with a tea kettle, drawing machines, and repairing marine instruments. At thirteen or fourteen years of age, he prepared a Barbary Organ ; at eighteen, at Glasgow, he learned to make mathematical instruments. He studied mechanics, physics, and chemistry under Doctor Black, examined Newcomen's engine, noticed its heat losses, and found that they proceeded partly from radiation from the cylinder and partly from the necessity of cooling the cylinder at each stroke of the piston.[1] He calculated this loss, which was equal to two quarters of the original heat ; and made many experiments with the object of avoiding it.

Thus he was filled with an ardent desire to reduce the heat losses observed in Newcomen's engine. This desire was working in him up to the day when the fertile idea of the condenser appeared. We may now learn the circumstances under which he made his discovery.

" It was in the Green of Glasgow. I had just gone to take a walk on a fine Sabbath afternoon. I had entered the Green by the gate at the foot of Charlotte Street—had passed the old washing house. I was thinking upon the engine . . . and gone as far as the

[1] Thurston, op. cit., p. 90.

Herd's House, when the idea came into my mind that as steam was an elastic body it would rush into a vacuum, and if a communication was made between the cylinder and an exhausted vessel, it would rush into it and might be there condensed without cooling the cylinder. I then saw that I must get quit of the condensed steam and injection water, if I used a jet as in Newcomen's engine. Two ways of doing this occurred to me. First the water might run off by a descending pipe, if an offlet could be got at a depth of 35 or 36 feet, and any air might be extracted by a small pump; the second was to make the pump large enough to extract both water and air . . . I had not walked further than the Golf House when the whole thing was arranged in my mind."

The invention was made. It remained to be completed by new experiments. On the next day, Watt tried his first condenser. He employed as the steam cylinder a large brass syringe. Other condensers were made each more perfect than the first . . . The results were constant; the invention was realized.

We may thus distinguish in the history of this discovery the three stages already considered in preceding inventions.

(a) Phase of conscious preparation; James Watt and an education directed towards science and machines.

(b) The phase of sudden revelation preceded by unconscious work. While on a walk, he suddenly thought of Newcomen's engine and the idea came to him that steam as an elastic fluid, would pass by itself into a vacuum.

(c) The phase of conscious invention. Watt examined the conditions to be realized and discussed the two possible methods.

2. *George Stephenson and the Locomotive*

George Stephenson was born at Wylam in Northumberland, on the 9th June, 1781, as the son of

N

a poor miner, and entered at ten years of age the mine in which his father was working. He thus came in contact with machines from his earliest years. At seventeen, he was driving the winding machine of which his father was fireman. As a child he had made engines of clay, and he now studied the engines of Newcomen and Watt, and drew them in order to be able to understand their mechanism better.

He married at an early age, and felt the need to educate himself in order to augment his means. We may bear in mind this influence of need.

We find him tending the ponies in a coal mine, then driving an engine at Montrose, in Scotland ; later, with the object of paying the debts of his father, he repaired a Newcomen engine.

Necessity brought him to perform another task. Fire broke out in his house and destroyed the cuckoo clock. Being a poor man, Stephenson could not employ a clockmaker ; in the same way he had taken engines apart to learn their mechanism, so he took his clock to pieces, cleaned it and put it together again. As a prelude to his inventions, this work gave him the reputation in the whole village as a clockmaker. At a glance he learnt his calling : He saw that the obstacle to the working of the clock was congealed oil, and put the clock on the stove " to cook it ".

He was more than a clockmaker. He became a machine doctor, and the director of a mine entrusted him with the repair of a pump which clever engineers had not been able to put in order.

The idea then came to him that instead of repairing machines he might make new ones. He was visiting the coal mines of Blackett at Wylam and those of Blenkisop at Leeds. He cried, " I think I could make a better machine than this."

Locomotives already existed, but they were noisy, only travelled six miles an hour, and consumed a great deal of coal. Combustion had to be more economical, the noise had to be reduced, and a greater speed had to be obtained.

Stephenson therefore first invented a blower which avoided noise and increased the tractive power.

At last, in 1829, a prize was offered to the inventor of a locomotive capable of drawing a heavy load and travelling at 10 miles an hour.

The desire of winning this prize stimulated George Stephenson. He built a railroad from Liverpool to Manchester. Five machines were tried. On the decisive day Stephenson's *Rocket* travelled the first time at 20 miles an hour, and the second time at 29.

Improvements were made; Robert Stephenson, the son of the inventor in England, Marc Seguin in France, produced more powerful machines. But the essentials had been discovered. George Stephenson had had predecessors; Joseph Cugnot in France, Oliver Evans in America, Trevethick and Vivian in England. But the two elements which make up the essentials of a railway, the steam locomotive and the iron railroad, were invented by George Stephenson.

Three points are to be noticed in the story of this invention.

(1) Conscious preparation was long and evident : the life among machines, the drawing of the machines, the taking them apart, were an initiation into other inventions.

(2) The final invention resulted from a number of observations and intermediate inventions.

(3) In these successive constructions there appears to have been no sudden inspiration. However, in a few cases, Stephenson showed rapid and true insight, and was inspired with the hope of improving on his predecessors. The unconscious is to be found not in an incubation which preceded a sudden revelation of novelty, but in the logical sequence which, from the observation of the first engine to the realization of the *Rocket*, had fashioned, as it were, the mind of the inventor

little by little. There were ideas suggested in the mine, ideas aroused every day by the sight of machines, various impressions resulting from the desire to satisfy, and from the knowledge stored in memory, and all these were factors which reacted one on the other, often without the knowledge of the inventor, and were finally expressed in his creation.

3. *The Bicycle, invented by Michaux*

The bicycle may be cited as an example because, like the locomotive, it was invented after similar apparatus had been tried : the *draisienne* had preceded the tricycle and the tricycle had suggested the idea of the bicycle. The facts are as follows :—

(*a*) In 1816, Baron Daris de Saverbrun invented the *draisienne* or velocipede. This machine consisted of a pair of wheels in tandem, of equal diameter, and joined by a wooden connecting-rod. The rider propelled the machine by touching his toes to the ground with long strides.

(*b*) The tricycle completed the first apparatus, but this cumberous vehicle only had a short life.

(*c*) In 1855, the saddler, Michaux, of Paris, had to repair a tricycle. He played with the tricycle : Instead of three wheels, he fixed only two, pushed the front wheel with his feet, tried to move forward, fell, tried again, and finished by being able to keep his balance. The machine, when once started, seemed to go by itself. Up till then, he had put his foot on the ground in order to push the apparatus forward. He conceived the idea of adding wooden pedals to avoid touching the ground ; the wood was then replaced by iron, other improvements followed, and cycling took its present form.

We see the passage from one stage to another, from a complicated apparatus to a simple one, suggested little by little, by experience. We find unconscious work in this progressive inspiration as regards the details of construction. An experimental logic directs inventors, co-ordinates results, without their having at first an exact notion of the direction in which they are going.

IV. THE PATTERN LOOM

A multiplicity of invention co-ordinated with a view to a great and final invention is to be found in the magnificent work of Jacquard (1762–1834), the inventor of the pattern loom.

(a) The Beginning : A variety of Trades

Jacquard was born at Lyons on the 17th July, 1762, and was initiated into his future trade by his parents. His father, Jean-Charles Jacquard, was a foreman weaver of gold, silver, and silk brocade. His mother, Antoinette Rive, was a reader of designs. He early showed a lively taste for. all kinds of mechanism, and amused himself by constructing models of machines, towers, and churches remarkable for the exactness of their proportion.

He was soon set to bookbinding, and made new tools for the printers and cutlers. In this way he grew up in the midst of fabrics, and machines, and had experience of a variety of trades. He must thus have collected a great deal of knowledge quite unconsciously.

(b) First Invention

He had already, in 1790, thought out a mechanism for improving the loom. He made a study of the simple loom ; he worked with a view to eliminating the drawing of the lashes by hand.

Then came the Terror. In 1793, he was fighting, resisting the oppressors at Lyons, was obliged to flee, joined the regiment of Rhone et Loire with his son, who was killed. This stimulated him still more to invent, for, with his wife, he had to plait straw for making hats in order to live. Need made him ingenious.

182 UNCONSCIOUS IN THE SCIENCES

He attempted to manufacture new stuffs by more economical methods; in 1807, he made a model of a new loom for avoiding the drawing of the lashes and presented it to the Industrial Exhibition. He was rewarded by a bronze medal " for having eliminated a workman in the manufacture of brocade by inventing a mechanism to replace him ". Before his time, in fact, all the threads which had to be lifted together in order to form designs on brocade were lifted by cords, pulled by a child, the draw boy, when the weaver gave the sign. In the Jacquard apparatus this system is replaced by the movement of a single pedal which the operator works himself.

In 1802 this machine was despatched to Paris and examined at the Conservatoire des Arts et Métiers. Carnot congratulated the inventor : " You, he said to him, have done the impossible : you have made a knot with a stretched thread." He obtained patents for his invention in December, 1802.

(c) Second Invention : The manufacture of net

At this moment the desire to win a prize stimulated Jacquard's activity. In England the Society of Arts offered a reward for the inventor of a loom for weaving net. Jacquard, called by Carnot, worked at it in Paris, under the direction of Molard, and had his invention adopted at Lyons.

Jacquard's invention was thus two-fold; he constructed a loom to weave net, and invented the mechanism necessary to abolish drawing the cords by hand. In this work he was inspired by the labours of his predecessors : Vaucanson had invented the simple hand loom ; La Selle had perfected it by adding hooks. Jacquard replaced the work of the draw boy by a suitable mechanism.

It only remained to make the working of the hooks more regular by the use of springs. The idea was suggested by a workman, Arnaud, and was carried out by another workman, Breton, under Jacquard's direction. Thus, in constructing his masterpiece, the inventor made use, not only of his own previous discoveries, but also the suggestions of others.

(d) *The Psychological Process in the case of this Invention*

(1) Its author was prepared for it unconsciously by an environment in which the necessities of existence obliged him to work : the example of his father and mother, the sight of machines, and of textiles, etc.

(2) The author was introduced to inventions, in more distant sense, by the manufacture of tools for cutlers and printers. We may note this without stressing its importance. A miniature invention paves the way for a larger one, as was the case with George Stephenson.

(3) Urged on by the necessity for assisting his family, and also by a desire for fame, Jacquard made two inventions : the net loom and the mechanism which supersedes the draw boy. Consider the latter. The inventor had seen the boy whose duty it was to draw the cords which produce the designs in brocades ; he pitied him. Gradually, the desire to replace him by a mechanism awoke in his mind associations of ideas relating to the end he was aiming at. This was apparently a long and laborious task, without any flashes of inspiration ; at least, the author has not left us any confidences on this point. Hence, it is in these combinations of ideas by the sight of a child and a machine, and also in the relation between past inventions and the final one, that the unconscious exerted an influence in Jacquard's work.[1]

---

[1] Fortis, *Étude historique de Jacquard*, Paris, 1840 ; *Nouvelle Biographie générale*, by F. Didot, vol. xxv, pp. 212, 213, 214 ; *Memoires de l'Académie*, years 1801, 1806.

V. BORING MACHINES USED FOR DRIVING THE TUNNEL
THROUGH THE ALPS

Jacquard's invention took place at two separate times. We now come to a still more complex matter, the machines employed for driving the tunnel through the Alps, wrongly called the Mont Cenis tunnel, since it passes 27 kilometres to the west of this mountain. These machines were the result of five successive inventions produced by engineers who succeeded one another in carrying on the idea. These were conscious of the result aimed at, but were unconscious of the new procedure which was capable, after each failure, of reaching final triumph.

(a) Medail's idea

The first idea of this enormous tunnel was due to Medail, of Bardonneche. The fact struck him ; in this part of the Alps the chain is not very broad, and the passes which give access from La Maurienne in the valley of Oulx are very numerous. The idea came to him one day that the Alps could be pierced in this region. For more than twenty years he continued his exploration. They confirmed his first conviction. He communicated his ideas to others, and, before his death, he was able to see a commission working on the question.

But it was a matter of making an opening of 30 kilometres length in the mountains 1,600 metres high. Ordinary means would require at least 36 years of work and this fact at first led to the proposal being rejected.

(b) The Mauss Machine, 1849

The Belgian engineer, Mauss, fortunately came to the assistance of the commission and offered it in 1849 a machine that he had invented. In this apparatus the connection between the motor and the drill had to be made by very long belts, but in this long gallery the belts could not be brought to a sufficient tension.

Furthermore, the apparatus had no power to renew the vitiated air. Although it was excellent for boring rock, this machine, which was operated by hydraulic power, did not combine in itself the necessary qualities for boring so long a tunnel. The only result of this trial was a psychological one. The problem had been stated and the idea would be taken up again on the first occasion.

(c) Colladon's Machine, 1855

In 1855 Colladon, of Geneva, offered the commission, which continued in existence, a compressed-air motor which he had invented. This time, transmission of power and ventilation of the shaft were combined, which was a result unobtainable by Mauss' method. The problem was now how to obtain compressed air in great quantities. The means existing at that time were considered to be inadequate. A third constructor, Bartlett, then appeared.

(d) Bartlett's Machine

This machine solved the problem ; it was a horizontal steam locomobile, but its motive power could not be applied in tunnels.

(e) The Hydraulic Compressor

At this point the idea arose of combining the three systems. The new machine would be able to produce sufficient power to bore clear, and aerate the tunnel as the excavations proceeded. Three Sardinian engineers, Grandis, Grattoni and Sommeiller, built for this purpose the hydraulic compressor. A fall of water of 20 metres operated the apparatus ; the air was compressed to six atmospheres, and effected at once the ventilation of the tunnel, the drilling of the rock, and the clearing away of the debris produced by blasting.

(f) *Vallaury and Buguet's Apparatus*

Nevertheless, the debris caused by blasting was an inconvenience. Two engineers, Vallaury and Buguet, conceived the idea of getting rid of blasting, they made a new and powerful apparatus for attacking the rock directly without the help of powder.

SUMMARY AND CONCLUSIONS

This inquiry into the domain of technology has brought us the following results.

(1) Technical inventions are as innumerable as human desires, and arise in response to these desires or needs.

(2) Conscious preparation is ordinarily long and complex. Almost all inventors in this domain are in close touch with their contemporaries or predecessors ; they construct machines analagous to other machines, and work ceaselessly to perfect them. All the inventors studied have spent years working at the construction of machines already existing and criticizing their defects. This preparation was often unconscious, since the inventors in question were not yet aiming definitely at their discovery, but often conscious as regards the repeated attempts to gain success.

(3) The finished invention is the work of the creative imagination, that is to say the image formed as the result of the work of synthesis, the details of which remain unknown. The unconscious suggests associations, substitutions, and other syntheses of ideas absorbed from the study of other machines.

(4) There remains the work of verification. This is often a conscious mental process to begin with, the idea being pictured as operating in the mind. There follows the test of the actual machine. This verification is obviously conscious. In technology, invention is progressive ; the machine is built wheel by wheel ; the

apparatus is arranged piece by piece. A machine is, in this respect, the invention which best expresses the intellectual mechanism which brings about its realization. Composed as it is of parts which act upon and drive one another, it is the material model of that interplay of feelings and thoughts of consciousness and the unconscious which, as we shall see in the second part of this study, is found in the intellectual origin of all inventions.

CHAPTER VII

COMPARISON OF THE GENERAL RESULTS OF THIS INQUIRY

Phenomena of feeling : in mathematics, physics, biology, moral sciences, in technology—Conscious intellectual phenomena : preparation, sudden intuition, verification—Unconscious intellectual facts : knowledge in general and in the various sciences.

I. PHENOMENA OF FEELING

WE find an affective element in all sensation and all feeling. Also, in perception, the psychological antecedent is sensual, since it is the sensation itself. In judgment, an affective element is again found, for we pass from the sensation to the image before rising from the image to the idea.

(*a*) In mathematics, Pascal's researches were governed by an ardent desire for knowledge ; the desire for fame and the need of money stimulated Ampère ; the æsthetic sentiment, love of order, inspired Poincaré ; the desire to find a demonstration proving both for the reason and for the eyes caused me to discover a new method of establishing the theorem that the sum of the angles of a triangle are equal to two right angles.

(*b*) In physics we have found a lively desire, an imperious need, almost a passion for success in the case of the inventors we have studied.

(*c*) In biology Claude Bernard tells us that feeling takes the initiative. Feeling for beauty and taste for symmetry inspired Pascal, while Darwin was animated by the desire to generalize his observations. In the moral sciences, a lively desire and thirst for truth inspired the philosophers whom we have discussed.

(*d*) Finally, in technology the vaiety of human desires corresponds to the multitude of machines.

(e) In all sciences as in the case of all inventions, immense joy follows discovery. This took the form of a mystical exaltation in the case of Kepler, Gutenberg, and Descartes ; of an ecstasy produced by the unveiling of a new order in the case of Newton, Pasteur, and Ampère. In all these cases it was an enthusiasm evoked by an original vision of rational beauty.

II. Conscious Intellectual Phenomena

Previous analysis allows us to divide these into three : Conscious preparation, sudden intuition of the generative idea of the invention, and conscious verification.

(a) Conscious preparation is more or less long. All inventors whom we have studied have spent much time, often from their infancy, in absorbing and studying their subjects and allied fields of knowledge. In the case of all, particularly in the field of mathematics and physics, there is a discontinuity between the work of research and the appearance of the new idea. In the case of all of them, particularly in that of biology and technology, we are struck with the variety of researches motivated by changes in the original hypothesis. In all cases, finally, we have seen the close connection between inventions ; each one realized, itself the result of analogy to the previous conception, prepares for a new one which is an improvement on the first. Hence every new designer studies his predecessors. Since bold creation is only possible by the assimilation of elements borrowed from various scientists, geniuses such as Ampère and Pasteur prepare for invention by the most general and varied culture.

(b) We now have the fertile idea, the discovery of the fundamental idea of the invention. The phenomenon is conscious ; it is a sort of vision or revelation. This does not happen in all cases in the same way. We can distinguish various degrees in the intensity of this manifestation. We have as it were a gamut of different keys in which the new idea is presented. We may classify them as follows in the order of the faculties concerned, and also in the order of their suddenness.

To begin with, we find the novelty in every *sensation*, this is its representative or significant element.

Equally, there is invention in a new *feeling*, the origin of which is not perceived ; Comte offered us a remarkable example of a transformation in invention produced through feeling.

The judgment of inference by which all *perception* is effected is likewise new ; the affirmation of this judgment is invention.

The act of *recognition* by which the *memory* precisifies the objects of its recollections is also invention.

The *imagination*, with its innumerable creations, resulting from manifold combinations produces as its invention the new image which it reveals.

In *judgment*, the affirmation of the suitability or unsuitability to the subject of a given attribute is a novelty, above all if the judgment is synthetic, for other attributes might be suitable.

In the ordinary *syllogism* and in all complete or incomplete *reasoning* it is not only the conclusion which is invented, it is also, and sometimes solely, a premise, the major or the minor, since, in response to a special psychical state, it is suggested so as to lead to a desired conclusion.

In general, the expression of an opinion or a new belief is an invention, since it is a thought, and every thought differs in some respects from every other thought and constitutes a true creation.

Now, sensations, feelings, perceptions, recollections, mental images, judgments, reasonings, and opinions are found in the various forms of intellectual activity. We have thus regarded invention in the most general sense. So far it is obscure, unmarked, generally indistinct, but none the less real, for it expresses that a new phenomenon has appeared in the mind. These productions are common to all minds and not reserved to those called inventors, but they are nevertheless the common heritage of the latter.

However, they are more than this ; let us consider psychologically those inventions which are special to inventors.

In the case of the great majority these take the form of the conception of an analogy or the first idea of an hypothesis covering a large number of facts. There is no element of well marked surprise or suddenness ; on the contrary the moment of conception is often hardly definite. The invention is the result of slow elaboration ; it arises without its point of contact with the logical antecedents being known. It is like a seed germinating and pushing its way through the ground without our being able to determine exactly the moment of its appearance. The hypothesis or new theory is found as if by chance in the mind, as the result of slow crystallization.

In the case of other inventors, the fertile intuition takes the form of sudden illumination, of a quick flash, of a vision. It seems as if the intuitive reason had grasped the truth, without the action of intermediate faculties.

We have seen that these two forms are to be found in all the sciences. All the same, the slow procedure of progressive revelation by analogy is particularly characteristic of physics, biology, and technology ; in these the hypothesis is modified little by little and the final conception of a general law is reached by successive approximations. On the other hand, the sudden vision which reveals the solution sought for is met with more particularly in the domain of mathematics and moral science. In the case of mathematics, conscious logic begins the syllogism, which is of a simple character, and it ends, after unconscious elaboration, in a conclusion as simple as the premises, and hence capable of appearing suddenly. As regards the psychologists and sociologists, we must note that the principle of one of their theories may be as simple and general as the major of a syllogism in mathematics; the difficulty is to find it. It is not therefore surprising that after a long period of minute research, the fundamental idea appears in its most general form by a sudden intuition.

(c) It remains for us to consider conscious verification. This is an experiment either in thought, that is to say a process of reasoning, or in the material world, which justifies the significant element of the sensation, the judgment of perception, the correctness of the imaginative product, the exactness of a simplified process of reasoning, the extent of an hypothesis and the extension of an analogy.

III. Unconscious Intellectual Facts

We may now group together all the facts which, as a result of our preceding analysis, we have found to be unconscious in some degree. We have grouped under this heading all mental or physical activity which escapes the clear view of consciousness. We thus include not only absolutely unconscious facts, but also those partially conscious, and even those the examination of which shows but a slight fringe of the unconscious.

In knowledge in general, we have found the unconscious in the latent judgment which allows sensations to be appreciated, and in the mental process resulting in the formation of various feelings. It explains the illusions of optics, judgments of size, and judgments of perception according to the theory of inference; it is the germ of ideas pre-existing in memory; it is the hidden force which produces in the imagination the elaboration of revery and dream, and also the uprising of ideas discussed in meditation; we find it in the judgment, which is the conclusion of a latent process of thought. Its slow rumination is responsible for the majors of syllogisms, various forms of hypothesis, and more generally of analogy. We owe to it our opinions, our beliefs and our doubts.

In the various sciences, we have seen the effects of this latent activity of the unconscious. There is no difficulty in admitting this activity when the fundamental idea of the invention is revealed suddenly in a flash ; there is so much difference between the new phenomenon and the preceding state, that we are driven to assume a mysterious activity in order to explain it. Certain philosophers, such as Desdouits and Rignano, have questioned the existence of unconsciousness in those moments when the mechanism of thought is obscure ; they do not think that there is an element of unconsciousness in sensation, in perception, in general reasoning, in analogies, etc. " In invention," says Rignano, " the idea passes from the potential condition to the actual condition by means of the effective tendency . . . in the potential state, it is neither conscious nor unconscious, it does not exist." [1] Others think that they have explained everything by regarding as the effects of habit a large number of psychical acts which are not perceived by the subject. The *potential state* and *habit* would thus be two notions which would allow us to dispense with recourse to the unconscious.

This appears to be rather replacing one term by another than giving a solution of the problem. Habit assumes a certain degree of unconsciousness ; it tends to reduce consciousness. This point is admitted by everyone. There is thus no incompatibility between our point of view and that of the psychologists named.

Furthermore, what is the potential state of an idea if it be not the equivalent of that idea in a hidden form ? For potential here is not simple possibility, which although possible, does not yet exist ; it is not a mere nothing. It is a being which already exists, although incomplete ; it awaits its perfection, its complements, its act. A block of marble is not a statue, but it already possesses an element of the statue ; it is a potential statue. We could not say that relative to the statue it is nothing at all. The energy of a stretched spring can be used to raise a weight; it therefore possesses actual energy. But when it is regarded in its stretched but immobile condition, we say that it has potential energy; the capacity to do work is in reserve, but it is not a simple possibility, it exists. In the same way before the act itself which arouses the recollection, there is a latent force in the memory which at the desired moment will set free the recollection. To say that this hidden energy is nothing at all because we do not see it, would be to admit that the recollection is produced out of nothing, and that we are dealing with a miracle. We must thus recognize that the recollection is there in a potential state. The same is true of the psychical antecedents, which, by their transformation, allow an analogy to be born. One thing is produced from two, or else these hidden elements, in the potential state, are nothing at all, in which case the anology is an effect without cause, an inadmissible product. If, however, the elements are a reality, the anology is explained: the effect is referred to a cause. But since this cause is hidden, and not perceived by me, I have the right to call it unconscious.

To sum up, Rignano, when he says that a potential state is nothing at all, is confusing pure possibility or non-repugnance of existence with the potential state of existence begun, but embryonic and incomplete.

Hence the distinction between the two forms under which invention appears, slow crystallization and sudden revelation, is without importance for our subject. It is a quantitative difference. We have to pass from the conscious logical antecedent of the invention to C, the generative idea of the invention, by way of B, which is the necessary unconscious intermediate, Whether C is manifested gradually and necessarily, or whether it is revealed in a sudden flash, B is equally necessary in both cases.

SECOND PART

GENESIS OF THE INVENTION UNDER THE INFLUENCE OF THE UNCONSCIOUS

CHAPTER I

THEORY OF INTEGRAL KNOWLEDGE

Statement of the question—Sensation, feeling, and thought in knowledge—Feeling, thought, and tendency in knowledge—Intuition and reasoning in knowledge—Conscious and unconscious factors—The relative position and importance of feeling, intuition, reasoning, activity, consciousness, and the unconscious in all intellectual construction.

1. *Statement of the question*

UNDER integral knowledge we understand the whole process of knowledge, that is to say, the sum of all psychical activities which combine in the great work of invention. Invention is the result of numerous conscious and unconscious forces, and hence this theory of integral knowledge will be the account of all the forces necessary to explain the final result. It will be a general view of the whole psychical ferment which results in the birth of an original work.

As we have said, invention is the highest point of knowledge, a culminating point attained by genius, but it is not qualitatively distinguishable from knowledge in general. Thus our theory of integral knowledge, although developed with a view to explaining invention, will still be quite general as an exclusively psychological theory.

We may state the question to be discussed. It is not a matter of fusing together, in the pages that follow, the concepts of feeling, intelligence, will, consciousness, and the unconscious. The phenomena of feeling are one thing, the intellectual phenomena are another, the voluntary phenomena yet another. On the other hand the conscious fact, clearly perceived by the subject, remains very distinct for us as compared with an unconscious, sub-conscious, or half-conscious fact, which to some extent is a mystery for our minds. But it does not follow that, because these two elements are logically different, they are in fact separated in mental activity. We propose to show that synchronism and synergy exist in every act of knowledge. Hence, taking the different facts two by two before uniting them in a final synthesis we shall examine successively in the mechanism of knowledge :—

(1) The co-existence of feeling or sensation, and thought.

(2) The union of feeling, thought, and the tendency to action.

(3) The alliance between intuition and reasoning.

(4) The succession, in these various phases of mental activity of consciousness and the unconscious.

(5) Finally, the place and relative importance of feeling, intuition, reasoning, activity, the unconscious, and consciousness, in all intellectual construction.

II. THE SENSATION, FEELING, AND THOUGHT IN KNOWLEDGE

In affirming the copenetration of sensible and intellectual factors in the mechanism of knowledge, we are echoing the opinion of a large number of distinguished writers and thinkers.

Alfred de Musset writes :—

" Ah ! frappe-toi le cœur : c'est là qu'est le génie ;
    C'est là qu'est la pitié, l'espérance et l'amour ;
    C'est là qu'est le rocher du désert de la vie,
        D'où les flots d'harmonie,
    Quand Moïse viendra, jailliront quelque jour ! "

On the other hand, who does not know the maxim of Vauvenargues : " Great thoughts come from the heart." Nothing could be more true, but is this the whole truth? Great thoughts are born of feeling. Why should not smaller thoughts, in a sense, have the same origin?

A psychologist who was also a doctor, Antonin Eymieu, replied to this question: " All thought, he writes, is mingled with sensation: that is why every idea in man stirs the appetite for the corresponding act. An angel has no sensations . . . in the case of man there are no pure sensations and no pure thoughts : He feels and thinks with his soul."

" The soul, which is a unity, is set in motion in its whole reality. Thought imbibes all its sensations and *vice versa* ; or if this metaphor be preferred, there is produced between them a sort of endosmose and exosmose and, as thoughts are always wrapped around by sensations, sensations are wrapped around by thoughts." [1]

Every idea tends to its own realization. Since " it is only efficacious to the degree in which it is mingled with feeling ", it only acts if it is felt. Hence every idea is more or less felt. More generally, all thought is enveloped in feeling.

But the reciprocal is also true. Fouillée tells us that : " all feeling envelopes ideas."

Joyau gives us a plausible reason for this. Ideas come either from experience or from the association which evokes them, or from the imagination which produces them by combination. Now, in the first case, present experience causes the appearance along with the sensation of the significant element, the germ of the perception, and therefore arouses the sensation and the idea at the same moment. In the same way, association by analogy, by contrast, or by transference, evokes the corresponding idea by virtue of the law of interest, that is to say by way of a feeling. Once more, the feeling heralds the idea. There remains the case of imaginative combination.

[1] Eymieu, *Le gouvernement de soi-même*, vol. i ; *Les grandes lois*, Paris, 1905, pp. 79–80.

Why does such a new combination, which produces an original idea, result from a preceding dissociation ? A choice has been necessary. The selection was decided by the hidden influence of interest or feeling. Further, the result of imaginative work is an idea presented in the form of an image. Now, as Godfernaux has shown, " the sensation and the image are identical in nature." [1]

Thus, in all three hypotheses quoted, feeling is not separated from thought. [2]

We may, however, go more deeply into the question, as Bain, Bergson, and Segond have done, and ask what it is which holds feeling and thought indissolubly together.

According to Bain, it is in a state of emotion that feeling constantly acts upon the intelligence to fertilize it : " In all these compositions (these creations of the mind), the directive power is an element of refined emotion, and this is the basis of all creative effort . . . The emotion must awaken the object, and the object the emotion . . . When an emotion has taken a powerful hold of the mind, nothing which disagrees with it can find a place, while the weakest link is sufficient to recall the circumstances which are in harmony with the dominant state."

From this it follows that " in minds most subject to emotion, the most purely intellectual links of association combine and change continually under the influence of feeling ".

Bergson goes more deeply than Bain, back to the source of feeling itself, life, to explain this permanent union between sensibility and intelligence : " The theory of knowledge and the theory of life are inseparable one from another." . . . On the other hand, " life is the continuation of an urge which is divided up among

---

[1] Godfernaux, *Le sentiment et la pensée et leurs principales applications psychologiques*, Paris, 1894, p. 132.

[2] Cf. Joyau, *De l'invention dans les arts, dans les sciences*, Paris, 1879, *passim*.

divergent lines of evolution." As a consequence of creative evolution, "reality appears to us like an uninterrupted fountain of new experiences." Intelligence "causes new ideas to arise from new feelings ".[1]

The intelligence itself, for M. Bergson "is the shrinkage by condensation of a vaster power, life itself." If we only consider the phenomenon of perception, "it is a selection, it eliminates what does not interest the body," that is to say feeling—which he calls vital instinct or interest, is at the base of knowledge.[2]

As a result of the flexibility introduced into the mind by sensibility, "the intelligence, says Segond, is sympathy with everything ; intelligence is a life." [3]

This is also the opinion of Dwelshauvers, in the work which we have frequently quoted :—

" Before expressing a thought, we have a confused feeling of it ; our consciousness seems distended as it were by the ideas which are about to well up ; this state is not clear ; it is emotive."

On this question, Maine de Biran is still more explicit. He distinguishes internal affective perception from external affective impression. Speaking of the latter, which result from the immediate action of objects on the senses, he decomposes them into two elements, one affective, the other perceptive. He sees two phases in the total impression : at the first moment, the affective part and the perceptive part are in equilibrium. Then the second phase commences : the affective part is degraded, while the perceptive part becomes prominent. He verifies this co-existence and these variations in respect of the impressions of each of the five senses.[4] When he passes from perception to reasoning he finds

[1] Bergson (H.), *L'évolution créatrice*, Paris, 1921.
[2] Bergson (H.), *Matière et memoire*, p. 255.
[3] Segond, *Intuition et amitié*, p. 67.
[4] Maine de Biran, *Memoire sur les perceptions obscures*, Paris, 1920, *passim*.

again this simultaneity of feeling and thought : " A
certain higher instinct. a certain way of feeling, proper
to the personality of each of us, constitutes the active
part of reasoning.[1]

We may also hear what Rignano says concerning
this element of feeling in discursive logic. He explains
attention, reflection, coherence, the critical spirit, the
imagination, abstraction, the synthetic spirit, the
analytical spirit, and the reason, by affective tendencies.
These are desires or needs which drive the organism
towards " physiological invariability " ;   they are
mnemonic tendencies which reappear in all intellectual
operations, because they determine the aim and inspire
the conclusion. The following is the essential passage in
which his doctrine is characterized : " A happy idea
comes from a selection among an overproduction
of thought-of acts. If, as the result of affective choice,
the idea, which has been raised to the state of consciousness is maintained before the mind, reasoning
has a teleological direction : affectivity gives it coherent
thought." [2]   Thus Rignano believes that feeling plays
the part of a cement for ideas.

Let us take Herbart. His intellectualist doctrine
of emotion completes and modifies that of several of his
predecessors. The Stoics, before Herbart, made happiness
or unhappiness depend on the opinion which we have
of things : " What disturbs men, says Epictetus, is
not things, but the opinion which they form of things."
Leibniz says that : " Pleasure is a feeling of perfection,
and pain a feeling of imperfection, provided that it be
sufficient for us to perceive it." [3]   Wolf assigns a similar
cause to the same feeling : " A judgment which we make
on our own perfection." Herbart corrects these opinions
by making our feelings derive from " the agreement or
disagreement of our representations ", just as the musical

---

[1] Paliard, *Le raisonnement selon M. de Biran*, Paris, 1925, p. 196.
[2] Rignano, *Psychologie du raisonnement*, p. 127.
[3] *Nouveaux Essais*, ch. xx.

harmonies and discords come from the gamut itself. Here representations are the causes of emotion; they are not simply their accompaniment. We may simply lay hold of this fact : they are so called up and coexist for a moment, while remaining quite distinct.

Wundt is the philosopher who has considered most thoroughly the correspondence between feeling and thought. He calls " representation " every image produced in the consciousness by any object whatsoever. If the object is real, this representation becomes perception. He regards feelings as resulting principally " from the relations between representations in time and space ". As a result of this relation, " the duration of sensations depends upon the tone of the feeling which accompany them," the tone itself being influenced by its association with familiar representations. Kant had seen in feeling " the product of obscure or unconscious knowledge ". Wundt is not far from sharing this opinion when he formulates his thought as follows : " Feeling must always rest upon a procedure of unconscious conclusions by which the modification of our internal state provoked by sensations or representations, is determined as being a subjective modification.[1]

Is not this Wolf's " intuitive knowledge ", Kant's " obscure knowledge ", Hegel's " confused knowledge " ? When Godfernaux writes : " Tendency is known as emotion," [1] he also sees in the phenomenon of emotion a primordial stage of knowledge. Finally, Grote seems to state the same idea when he says : " feeling is the conscious product of an unconscious estimate of certain relations." Here, as in the opinion of Wundt, there is an intellectual operation, which is unconscious, and a sensible operation, which is conscious, and derived from the first.

In spite of the diversity of the point of departure these opinions agree in uniting a feeling and a thought

[1] Op. cit., p. 133.

in the same subjective state. Hence all of them are true up to a certain point, since what they state agrees with the facts.

Let us consider the question more closely and examine one of the facts in detail. I am shown a flag and I immediately recognize the three French colours. What passes in my mind ? A three-fold operation : (1) An unconscious judgment, which is the cause of my emotion, a judgment which has rendered possible the recognition of the national flag ; a necessary judgment, otherwise my emotion would be without a cause, but an unconscious one, since nothing tells me that I made it before my feeling is born. (2) A conscious feeling, since it was an emotion which I am conscious of, a feeling which, in certain cases, will be replaced by a vague sensation, but which always exists at the threshold of every perception. (3) A conscious judgment, the perception of that significant element which we discovered when analysing the mechanism of sensation and perception, a judgment which is explicit and clear, for I immediately recognize the national flag from the three colours. But we must note that the two first operations required by logic are combined psychologically to one only : the conscious feeling is welded to the unconscious judgment. Together, in their synthetic unity, they constitute a vague, confused, synthetic knowledge which might be called the *felt* knowledge. The third operation is clear, distinct, analytical knowledge ; it may be described as perceived knowledge. Hence, in these three operations, which are reduced to two, there is knowledge, a knowledge of two degrees : the first is inherent in the feeling, the second in the perception. On the other hand, in the first degree, we have found the unconscious and consciousness : The unconscious in the obscure judgment which serves as the substratum for feeling ; and consciousness, either in the feeling itself, or in the judgment of perception which follows it. This distinction will be of capital importance to the further

consequences which we shall draw from this first con-
frontation of feeling and thought. Since this analysis
applies to any knowledge whatsoever, the distinction
resulting from it may also be regarded as general.

III. FEELING, THOUGHT AND TENDENCY TO ACTION IN KNOWLEDGE

Feeling and knowledge, as living phenomena, tend
towards activity. They obey a fundamental law of
psychology, the law of systematic association, thus
formulated by Paulhan : " Every phenomenon produced
is the result of a systematic association of simpler
elements, and tends to cause the appearance of other
elements which can be associated with it and concur
towards a common end." [1]

(a) This tendency is a fact

This tendency to activity is characterized by Bain
as the necessary condition of all invention : it is not
by superior intellectual power, but by expending unusual
activity that a man makes discoveries.[2]

The sensation and the image are already simple
movements. Further, says Godfernaux : " Thought
in the case of the majority of individuals is predominantly
composed of motive elements . . . Now these movements in a nascent state, which reproduce the real
movements by which the tendency seeks to satisfy
itself, are known under the form of associations of ideas.
Thinking is associating, and associating is acting."
But in what sense ? Does conscious thought necessarily
pass on to action ? No, for the underlying tendency,
the basis of mental activity, may be in conflict, either
with another tendency, of with a group of tendencies

---

[1] Paulhan, *L'activite mentale et les éléments de l'esprit*, Paris, 1889,
p. 216.
[2] Bain, op. cit., p. 477

which act by inhibition.   In this case, we shall actually distinguish a moment, however short it may be, at which conscious thought remains in a state of suspension, resulting from the opposition of two antagonistic tendencies.   But then what does the mental representation become ?   With these two divergent drives, it is the result of two equal and contrary forces.   This result is zero.   The actual activity is thus zero.   However, the two tendencies have kept their character of forces. When the moment of equilibrium is broken, activity reappears.   That is how " mental representation is only a retarded activity ;   consciousness, says Godfernaux, interprets the preparation of activities which are actually suspended ".   We have a clear idea of it when the consciousness, affected by an increased coefficient of attention, maintains the mind in a kind of expectant condition, a condition of arrested activity.[1]

But this suspense is full of promise.   After the moment of preparation, there comes the moment of production : " the fertile thought, says Le Roy, is the thought which has become action."[2]

(b)   *In this tendency, feeling is a necessity*

The thought thus passes sooner or later into action ; action prolongs it, expands it, completes it.   But one condition is requisite : feeling.   There is correlation, between thought, feeling and action :—

" In order that a conscious being may be forced to act, says Dwelshauvers, it is necessary that he should have a desire, or more exactly, an effective state which sustains action."

Ribot, also writes as follows : " An idea does not act unless it is felt, unless it awakens tendencies, that is to say motive elements."

---

[1] Godfernaux, op. cit., pp. 141 et seq.

[2] L. Roy, " La logique de l'invention," *Revue de metaphysique et de morale*, 1905, pp. 193–223.

Maine de Biran extends this active influence to the whole field of deductive work : " A certain higher instinct, a certain way of feeling proper to the personality of each of us, constitutes the active part of reasoning." [1]

(c) The mode of this activity

We thus know that feeling is the necessary support of mental activity. Regarding the manner in which this co-operation takes place, Fouillée says :—

" To enjoy or to suffer, is to feel oneself living more or less . . . Pleasure is not potential force, it is the transformation of this force into living force, which causes pleasure . . . Pleasure is linked with the most intense vital activity possible." Now life is the total of the forces which resist death. Pleasure is thus a victory, pain a defeat. Thus, ideas may be forces unceasingly in relation with life and true functions of this life ; mental states must have an internal effectiveness and an external effectiveness." But the will presides over the activity. Hence, " ideas are formed, not only of thought, but of will." [2]

Fouillée thus regards ideas as effective, since they are forces, as closely linked with life ; and the sad or joyous which accompanies them appears as a minus or plus of life, as the tonality of life.

Rignano and Fouillée meet on common ground in this matter. For Rignano, in fact, pleasure is the revivification of vital energy, pain a state of depression of this energy." Consequently, feeling in one form or another certainly plays the part of a measure of life. [3]

(d) Its creative progress

This mental activity is susceptible of a great number of degrees, and is progressive. " Every instant of life,

[1] Paliard, op. cit., p. 196.
[2] *Psychologie des idées-forces*, p. 61.
[3] Rignano, op. cit., p. 35.

says Bergson, is original, that is to say different from every other, and includes an element of invention. We create ourselves continually . . . existence consists in changing, changing in ripening, ripening in creating oneself indefinitely."[1] Thus, adds Segond, "life transcends itself continually by its own invention . . . The real progress of the living being is an incessant creation."[2]

(e) *Reason for the copenetration of idea, feeling and activity*

Hitherto we have not found the deeper motive which links together thought, feeling and activity. These elements of the mind collaborate, but in unequal degrees. What relationship governs these variations ?

Is it sufficient to say, with Souriau, that " thanks to moral mimicry, we have a natural tendency to make ourselves like the objects of our contemplation ? " No ; for to state this tendency is not to explain it ; to derive it from mimicry is not to account for this urge to imitation.[3]

It will be said : " The idea tends towards its own realization ; now feeling presents the future act as good ; feeling is thus the intermediary between the act and its realization. That is why the repeated accomplishment of an act, by suggesting the idea of itself arouses little by little the feeling which is the normal link between a given idea and its execution."[4]

This certainly explains the connection between feeling and idea by the connection of both of them with the activity which crowns them. But I am seeking for the reason of this active tendency and the motive of this collaboration.

[1] Op. cit., p. 8.
[2] Segond, *L'intuition bergsonienne*, pp. 57, 74.
[3] Souriau, *La suggestion dans l'art*, p. 243.
[4] Eymieu, op. cit., p. 207.

Hoffding does not advance matters when, in order to elucidate the variable tonalities of intellectual and emotive phenomena, he distinguishes two stages in their comparative degree : if the intellectual element is dominant, we have a feeling ; if the sensible element is preponderant, an emotion. In the first case, if the intellectual element grows, the feeling evolves and tends to become knowledge ; in the second case, on the contrary, knowledge tends to vanish and the emotion is discharged in a definite act, or is changed into purposeless agitation.

This comparative study of the two elements, the intellectual and the sensible, does not touch the fundamental question : why, in this play of life, do we have this release of the idea, the feeling, and the act ?

Paulhan, without solving the question, brings into the debate the elements of the solution. He starts from the principle that every phenomenon of consciousness is accompanied by a physiological phenomenon, that is to say by a phenomenon connected with the nervous system. On the other hand, he defines *tendency* as a certain activity of the nervous centres. Hence an arrested tendency is a reflex act which cannot reach the goal towards which it tended. Now every affective state is accompanied by a tendency, and forms part of a series, the termination of which is movement. It is like a force associated with another force, the tendency ; these two forces have a result assumed to be constant. But if we arrest the tendency, the affected phenomenon gains what the tendency loses : It is *reinforced*. In practice, therefore, a well-characterized affective phenomenon marks the arrest of a tendency ; it indicates a want of co-ordination, it is due to an imperfect functioning of the mind. More generally, since there is sensibility in all consciousness, " every psychical fact is a tendency, and every conscious fact the arrest of this tendency." In short, sensibility and activity are the inverse of one another ; consciousness is not produced unless the psychical forces are in some degree

P

divided. Consciousness and the affective state thus coincide with a greater or less disturbance of the organism. They are due to the fact that a considerable quantity of nervous force is set into activity in a systematic manner. The psychical force has been set free in the nervous centres. But the tendency is arrested ; hence the force can no longer be expended. The result is emotion. This affective state is therefore a derivative of the force destined for activity. Just as electrical energy may be dissipated in heat and in mechanical work, so may vital force be expended in emotion and in movement. When the affective phenomenon is increased, the active phenomenon is diminished, in such a way as to leave the vital energy constant.

This explanation is ingenious. It is justified by the fact when we are dealing with emotions properly so called. Great joy does in fact arise from surprise, from good news received unexpectedly ; here we have an arrest of the tendency. In the same way, forbidden fruit is attractive, for the intensity of the desire come. precisely from the fact that it is practically unrealizable. In a general way, the remark of the poet Corneille remains true : " Et le désir s'accroit, quand l'effet se recule."

But we must notice that this phenomenon is only produced quite clearly when we are dealing with shock emotion, above all, when these emotions are caused by the impossibility of satisfying a tendency. But it is but slightly apparent if the fact of sensibility is a moderate feeling. However, if it is the feeling that supports the activity, as Paulhan recognizes, there is not necessarily an antagonism between the activity considered in the tendency, and the affective state. This opposition, which is very real when the realization of a desire is prevented, does not exist if the feeling agrees with the tendency. Rather, the activity will be the more intense, the more excited the sensibility by which it is inspired. The distinction established by

Paulhan between arrested tendency and non-arrested tendency calls for correction, and does not suffice to explain the general correlation between thought, feeling and activity.

(f) Proposed theory : vital synergy

Taking into account the most recent physiological investigation, let us first of all see how we are to understand the three phases of this psychological mechanism.

Biology teaches us that unicellular organisms, amœbas, rhizopods, leucocytes, seek the elements necessary for their life by selection and movement appropriate to this end. They thus have *sensibility* and *motile activity*; in their case, "the useful act follows perception of the need." Furthermore, these cells have a *memory*, since "successive impressions of the same order which they experience leave behind in them an imprint, as it were, of their passage, and from this results more and more easy reproduction of the original act."[1] These cells, which are the offspring of a single cell, are classified according to the part they play. Direction belongs to nerve cells or *neurons*, which are capable of sensibility. An impression occurs : it is received in a neuron, and transmitted from neighbour to neighbour along the whole chain of other neurons. As a result of cellular memory, the various neurons have registered their impressions. These impressions are translated into mechanical reaction. Now the organism contains almost six hundred millions of neurons. We thus have an immense army of cells in relation with one another, and remembering acts already accomplished ; their concerted action will thus release the corresponding act. Every living organism is characterized by the same mechanism. But man, more perfected, and gifted with a better memory, succeeds in

---

[1] Renaut, *Le Neurone et la memoire cellulaire*, pp. 11, 29.

carrying out acts corresponding to ideas suggested to him. Thus the search for elements necessary to life has been directed by sensibilities ; memory of the neurons represents elementary knowledge ; movement is the result of activity ; in short, sensibility, intelligence and activity find their ultimate reason in a biological necessity.

This is stating that part of the truth which is contained in the doctrines of Bergson, Rignano and Fouillée, but an explanation in terms of life is teleological explanation. Our opinions on this question, making use of Eymieu's ideas, completing or modifying them in certain points, are as follows :—

The idea, the feeling and the act constitute three moments of vital energy.

The living being is made to fulfil its end ; this goal is presented to him by the idea, the goal appears adequate and good through feeling ; consciously or unconsciously, the goal is sought by tendency.

Let us pause at the phase of the *idea.*

Vital energy crosses the threshold of consciousness. It is the revelation made to the ego of an external object, the impression of an image of this object. Now I am made up of a body and a mind, I am an incorporated soul. My idea will thus be the contact of the external world with the body and with the mind. But this relation with matter operates in space ; it has extension : it is sensation. This contact is conscious through the instrumentality of the mind. Now the mind is in contact with matter, with sensation, and borrows from it all that can be abstracted from it. This is thought.

We now come to the phase of *feeling.* This idea, which is born of sensation, meets other ideas, born of other sensations. Actions and reactions result, which act upon the unconscious region of the mind in order to draw from it the eddies of other actions and reactions. These are forces which harmonize or do not harmonize, drives which agree or disagree, elements which are adapted or are not adapted to synthesis. This action and this reaction, which constitutes an agreement or disagreement of the old existing ego with the new ego coming into existence, is *feeling*. The third phase then commences for the vital energy. It is that of the active *tendency*. This is a reaction of the ego upon the external world. The idea has given the tendency direction; feeling has furnished it with the assistance of other tendencies. The resultant of these forces produces the act.

Let us compare these three moments of vital energy. They interpenetrate. Feeling is active in the idea, since the idea, as a subjective fact and by virtue of its agreement or disagreement with other subjective facts, will excite feeling. More precisely, the tendency includes the feeling, since it is the latter psychological phenomenon which has robbed it of its confused character. Finally, at a given moment, the tendency and the sentiment have been conscious. The consciousness is an observed fact, hence a piece of knowledge. Thus the idea, the feeling and the tendency are different forms of knowledge. Then just as the consciousness is only a mode, or form of being, of thought, feeling and tendency, in the same way the unconscious in its various degrees may be a mode of these three aspects of vital energy. Consciousness and the unconscious represent vital force perceived or not perceived, observed or not observed, clear or confused, but always real.

We thus conclude that thought, feeling and active tendency represent distant states, but only states or modes of existence of the same psychic energy or the same vital force. Each of these states is capable, without changing its nature, of being by turns conscious or unconscious.[1]

We shall make use of this conclusion in the last part of this chapter.

---

[1] Cf. Eymieu, op. cit., pp. 306–21.

IV. In all Knowledge there is Intuition and Reasoning

(a) Intuition

Since, up to a certain point, interpenetration of actions, feelings and thought takes place, let us consider two aspects contained in this thought: intuition and reasoning. Let us define their nature and distinguish their rightful place in mental life. It is obvious that if we cannot separate feeling and activity from thought in the realm of actual fact, we cannot separate them from the two forms of thought. There will thus be feeling and activity both in intuition and in reasoning. But what are these two psychical operations in relation to one another ? What are they first of all in themselves ?

Let us first take intuition. The meaning attributed to this word has been, not modified, but developed, at the same time as psychology itself.

Considered as an attribute of God, intuition is distinguished from discursive knowledge, long and patient, which is the attribute of man. St. Thomas Aquinas, an Aristotelian, and a qualified representative of scholasticism, states this distinction in the following terms.[1]

"*Divina cognitio non est inquisitiva : non per ratiocinationem causata, sed immaterialis cognitio rerum absque discursu.*"

Joseph de Maistre concludes from this text : " Science in God being an intuition, the more it has this character in man, the nearer it approaches to its model.[2]

It is this sense which has been retained by the theologians : intuition is God's supernatural knowledge, which is superior to natural knowledge. Applied to man, intuition is certain and spontaneous knowledge unaided by reason.

---

[1] Thomas Aquinas, *Adversus Gentes*, i, 92.
[2] *Soirées*, ii, xᵉ *entretien*.

The German philosophers Kant and Schelling give the word a significance which is somewhat different. For Kant, " intuition is external perception ; in its pure form it gives us notions of time and space ; in its empirical form it consists in the representations of the senses." As a follower of Kant, Schelling refers everything to the Absolute : " Intuition is the grasp of the Absolute in its identity by the intelligence."

The Scotch philosophers define this operation of the mind in a way which is nearer to the significance given to it in common language. " Intuition is an evident judgment, without reasoning and without reflection."

In a general way, we understand by this statement " beliefs and judgments anterior to all reflection ", or again, " sudden, spontaneous, indubitable knowledge, like that which sight gives us of objects."

Wundt gives intuition, in its relation to representation, a very limited sense : " Representation is the image produced by the object in consciousness." On the other hand, " perception is representation when it is concerned with the real object." Under these conditions, " Intuition is the activity of the consciousness which is directed towards grasping this object." [1]

Joyau, in the work we have already cited, insists upon the character of suddenness which we find in intuition : " It is the fertile hypothesis, the inspiration, the living light, the flash of lightning, the stroke of genius, the phenomenon which is as unforeseen as it is swift. It is a conception to which the series of reflections engrossing the scientist did not appear to be tending." [2]

We may now take Bergson. The author of *Creative Evolution* has made very considerable progress with the notion of intuition. It is through him that this operation of the mind, hitherto considered as an extraordinary means of knowledge, has become the indispensable complement of logical reasoning. Moreover, just as

[1] Op cit., ii, pp. 200–10.
[2] Op. cit., p. 110.

deduction is the business of the intelligence, intuition, a procedure which is different to that of deduction, is distinguished from true intellectual operation. This brings him to oppose intuition to intelligence; but this opposition is only apparent, since intuition and intelligence are derivatives of life.

Now life acts by an urge, which, says Segond, "recalls Leibniz's fulgurations and vital fountains." These fulgurations are continuous, the fountain play of novelties is uninterrupted. "Life is the continuation of one and the same urge, which is divided between the divergent lines of evolution." Practically, in the animal world, this original drive is instinct. The vital instinct in man, which is self-interested in its origin and unconscious in its first stage, becomes conscious and disinterested, becomes capable of reflection and, consequently, capable of enlarging its object indefinitely : it becomes *intuition*.

Bergsonian intuition is defined as "Instinct become disinterested, conscious of itself, capable of reflecting upon its object, and of enlarging it indefinitely." [1] This instinct is turned towards life, for intuition is "directed towards life"; and as "life is an effort to graft indeterminations", intuition is the first impulse towards these annexations; it seizes the invention as it springs up.

Segond has completed this notion of intuition and illuminated Bergson's thought. He defines it as "all knowledge which proves itself to be immediate and coincident with its object, that is to say, which introduces us into the latter and leaves us in it ". Now this object is of various kinds, and hence intuition will be of various kinds; when it is *sensible*, it unites us with objects in the external world, when it is *æsthetic* it becomes disinterested or playful contemplation ; when it is *affective* it is painful or joyous ; when it is *moral*, it becomes our personal work, we devote ourselves to it ; when it is *mystical* it is the divination of the profound

[1] Op. cit., p. 193.

meaning of things ; when it is *cosmic* it is a vision of the Universe in a fragment of the latter. In the case of woman, who is more attached to life than man and hence more instinctive and more primitive, " intuition is a fertile spirituality which results in an indefinable adroitness." Imitating as she does nature and life, " she has a sense of the occasion, and true sympathies." By virtue of a certain interpenetration of the senses, " she sees what she hears, she hears what she touches." [1]

What are we to retain of these various senses of the word intuition ? What is general and common to them, and what fits the everyday notion which we have of the intuitive man ? The intuitive mind is the one which divines : it seizes truth clearly and immediately without the assistance of proof ; it goes to the heart of truth by instinct, and hence intuition is instinctive knowledge ; it goes to it consciously, hence it is a conscious knowledge ; it moves towards it rapidly, and hence is a sudden grasping of the object ; it holds to this object with a certainty of not being deceived : sure of its conquest and greedy of progress, it reflects on its object, and, as Bergson says, it is capable of enlarging it indefinitely by grafting indeterminations on it. Thus, intuition will be for us immediate, certain and instinctive knowledge, the object of which is susceptible of vast development by means of reflection.

(b) Reason

Let us now consider reason. It consists in drawing from two judgments, admitted universal and necessary, a third judgment equally universal and necessary. Reasoning is, if we may make a useful comparison, crossing a brook too broad for a single stride in two steps by putting a stone in the middle. When it is deductive, it deduces the consequence from the principle. When it is inductive, it leads us from the particular to

[1] Segond, *Intuition et amitié*, Paris, 1919, pp. 5, 21, 23, 34.

the general, from the facts to the laws which govern them.

We will leave to logicians the business of discussing whether induction may be referred to deduction, or whether on the contrary, deduction may be reduced to induction, or, still further, whether deduction may be reduced to a construction.[1] In this psychological study, let us pause at the hidden motive-power which directs reasoning in some one particular sense, towards some one conclusion rather than another.

The answer to this appears immediately if, returning to the comparison which served above to illustrate the notion of reasoning, we ask the following questions : Why did the walker in order to cross the brook place the two necessary stones at one place in the brook rather than another ?　In order to arrive at the opposite bank at a spot determined in advance and well chosen.　It was a reason adapted to the end in view which guided him.

We claim to prove that the same is true of the origin of all reasoning.　On this question, we share up to a certain point the view of Rignano.　His theory is as follows :—

After having had recourse to affective tendencies to explain attention, reflection, coherence, the critical spirit, imagination, abstraction, the synthetic spirit and the analytical spirit, he builds up his empirical doctrine of reasoning as follows :—

" A happy idea comes from a selection, from an over-production of thought-of acts . . . If, as the result of affective choice, the idea which has been raised to the state of consciousness is maintained before the mind, reasoning has a teleological direction ; affectivity gives it coherent force."

" All reasoning is an experimental verification, a mental experiment, a series of experiments which are

---

[1] Cf. Binet, *Psychologie du raisonnement* ; Goblot, " Sur l'induction mathématique," *Rev. phil.*, 7 avril 1914 ; Williams James, *Principles of Psychology*, ch. xxii.

simply thought of . . . The logical process is reality put into action in imagination ; it is an experiment on our thoughts. Imagination makes these combinations with old memory-elements. The conclusion is a new mental vision."

Let us sum up the author's thought. A new analogy, suggested by affective tendencies, has been perceived by intuition. This will be the conclusion of the reasoning. But it is necessary to prove it. Imagination goes to work and forms combinations. One only will be retained : the one which fits the suggested conclusion. Being guided by the affective tendency, the reason is thus, by turns, an evocation of mnemonic elements, an exclusion of those which do not fit, and a selection of thoughts which can be utilized to reach the conclusion. When they are mentally realized, this three-fold operation and this choice of judgments appropriate to the end in view, constitute verification, and the reasoning itself is a succession of experiments which are simply thought of.[1]

This empirical theory of reasoning, while it is very ingenious, has only a partial foundation. Let us compare an experiment with a syllogism. In the first case, the conclusion suggested by hypothetical intuition is known : it is the law which we are wishing to establish ; this aim suggests the various forms of the trials that are made. In the second case, the conclusion has been inspired by the affective tendency ; it is vaguely known ; it is in order to prove it that a choice is made between the possible premises. There is thus an end in view just as there is in the varied aspects which are given to experience. In both cases, a verification is made either of the conclusion, or of the law which is anticipated. Up to this point, the method is the same in the two cases, that is to say, in the succession of phases in the psychological process. Only, however, we must note that, in experimenting, we remain observers, we await a concordance of phenomena which we are not free to

---

[1] Rignano, op. cit., pp. 117–70.

produce at will ; and if, as a result of critical examination, this conformity is found, the final conclusion will not be due solely to experience but will have been established by experience followed by a process of reasoning based upon this experience.

In reasoning, on the contrary, the mind is at the same time spectator and actor. As spectator it examines the validity of the premises ; as actor, it arranges the connection between the propositions, eliminates some of them if necessary, estimates the degree of demonstrative force, and supported by a sense of direct certainty, makes its way to the conclusion, which becomes evident without further control.

The difference between the two psychological procedures is thus manifest : experience by itself is insufficient. The mind requires two operations ; experience, and the criticism of this experience. Reasoning presents them to us bound up together ; in ordinary experience they are successive and not united. We may thus admit with Rignano that reasoning is " a series of experiences simply thought of ", if we add that these experiences are incited one by the other, as a result of the activity of the operator, who controls all the details as they are produced.

To this correction we must add another. An experiment is a sensible fact which interests several senses at once : sight, hearing, etc. Thus reasoning, in order to be experimental, should affect the senses in a certain way, and as it is distinguished from perception, which interests the external senses, it should bring into play the faculty corresponding to external perception, the imagination.[1]

Binet has understood this fact, and in this respect he has very successfully completed Rignano's theory : " The fundamental element of the mind is the image.

---

[1] Segond sees the essential nature of reasoning " In the power of invention, in the personal force of the imagination ". Cf. " L'activité intentionnelle de l'esprit " in the *Journal de psychologie*, 15 dec. 1925, p. 831.

Reasoning is an organization of images determined by the propriety of these images. It is sufficient for them to be called up. They then organize themselves and reasoning follows with the inevitability of a reflex.

How is this grouping produced ? " In external perception the images produced by the contact of objects form a whole which corresponds to the notion of a single object." Ordinary experience thus produces the appearance of such images. If reasoning is an experience in thought, it will therefore result, like perception, from the co-ordination of parallel images. And that is exactly what happens. Actions, sensations, and thoughts tend to reawaken those which resemble them. Hence each image is linked with the preceding one by those points which are common. We thus obtain, for the images a, b, c and d, various groupings such as abc, bcd, acd, etc. Reasoning thus becomes " the transition from a known fact to an unknown fact through the intermediary of a resemblance ". Hence three characters are common to perception and reasoning : (1) " They belong to mediate and indirect knowledge " ; (2) " They require the intervention of truths previously known and serving as premises " ; (3) " They presuppose the recognition of a similarity between the fact affirmed and the truth on which it rests." [1]

Let us now state our conclusions. As Rignano thinks, reasoning is a succession of experiences in thought. But it is more than this : it is a succession of experiments which the thinker calls up, and which he continually controls. In order to be a series of experiments, reasoning is also an association of images produced by other like associations, as Binet thinks. Since the affective tendency has provoked this grouping of images with a view to a conclusion felt in advance, reasoning is therefore a verification, and its procedure is teleological. But since rational control is actively exercised, rejecting one

[1] Binet, *La psychologie du raisonnement*, Paris, 1896, pp. 10, 82, 95.

premise and one image, and encouraging the appearance
of another proposition and another image, well conducted
reasoning is more than a succession of experiments,
more than a verification, it is a demonstration.   It is
under this aspect that we shall consider it in invention.

But reasoning is the essential operation of the
intelligence.   Let us pass from the act to the faculty.
Bergson has the credit for having well characterized
the origin and rôle of the intelligence.   We may sum up
his view.

" Vital activity divided as it grew " into two divergent
directions : *instinct*, which, when conscious, is intuition,
and *intelligence*.   They differ, not in degree, but in nature.
These two tendencies are mingled.   " Intelligence is
never found without traces of instinct.   Instinct is never
found but surrounded by a fringe of intelligence."
Intelligence treats everything mechanically ; " it   is
the faculty of manufacturing artificial objects."   Its
knowledge does not deal with things, but with relations,
not with matter, but with form.   As it leaves the hands
of nature, with manufacturing in view, its principal
object is the inorganic solid ; in decomposing and
recomposing matter, " it only imagines clearly discontinuity ; in order to attach itself to the actual or
future positions of an object, it can only imagine clearly
immobility."   It is characterized by the faculty " of
decomposing according to any law whatsoever, and
recomposing in any system whatsoever " ;   being
preoccupied with building up from given data, it allows
whatever is new to escape it, it rejects all creation, and
does not admit the unforeseeable.   At its ease in
manipulating inertia, " it is characterized by failure
to understand life." [1]

This analysis is well founded, provided we do not see
more in these characteristics of intelligence than preponderating tendencies.   For example, it is not exact
to state that intelligence can only imagine clearly

[1] *L'évolution créatrice*, xive, pp. 164–79.

immobility. If a mathematical student can understand more easily the equation $2x = 10$ than the function $y = 2x$, it is certainly true that it is because, in the first case, x is equal to five, which is a unique and constant reply, whereas in the second, x being given various values, y receives corresponding *variable* values.

In the case of the equation, the mind stops at a fixed quantity, in the case of the function, the intelligence has to picture to itself moving magnitudes. But we do not need to exaggerate the case. The intelligence understands the function with greater difficulty, but it does grasp it clearly and distinctly, since the intelligence " grasps the relationship between things ", as Bergson himself says, and since here to comprehend the idea of function is to comprehend a relationship of magnitude.

Having made this observation let us keep in mind above all the fact that the intelligence alone, operating on data, and rejecting the unforeseeable, is incapable of creation.

(c) *Intuition and Reasoning*

Since intellectual creations are innumerable and produced unceasingly, and since, on the other hand, intelligence or reasoning alone is incapable of producing them, they must be the result of the combined action of intuition and reasoning ; of intuition in their origin and of reasoning in their development.

This necessary co-operation between intuition and deduction has been affirmed by Schopenhauer :—

" There is no truth," he writes, " which could issue solely from a syllogism : the necessity for founding it on syllogisms is always relative, and even subjective. Since all proofs are syllogisms, the first care in regard to a new truth is not to seek a proof of it, but immediate evidence, and it is only in default of this, that we proceed provisionally to a demonstration. No science can be absolutely deductive, any more than one can build in the air ; all its proofs must bring us back to an intuition, which is not demonstrable."

A little further on, the same philosopher proves the generality of this statement :—

" Ultimate evidence, original evidence is an intuition, as its name indicates. Or rather, it is either empirical, or it rests on an *a priori* intuition of the conditions of the possibility of experience. In both cases, it only brings immanent and not transcendental knowledge. Every concept only exists and only has value by virtue of being in relation, no matter how distant, with an intuitive representation : what is true of concepts is true of the judgments which they have served to form, and also of all science."

Finally, Schopenhauer thus sums up his view :—

" Intuition—whether pure and *a priori*, as in mathematics, or *a posteriori* as in the other sciences—is the source of all truth and the foundation of all science . . . Judgments proceeding direct from intuition and founded on it as their only proof, are to science what the sun is to the world. It is from them that all light proceeds and everything that they have illuminated is capable of illuminating in its turn. To found immediately upon intuition the truth of these judgments, and to distinguish the foundations of science among the infinite variety of things, that is the work of the judgment properly so called.[1]

According to this philosopher, intuition is the basis of judgment. But reasoning is a chain of judgments ordered in respect of a final conclusion. Intuition is thus the foundation of all processes of reasoning ; it illuminates their birth, it directs their development. It is a lighthouse at the starting point, lighting up the ocean of science ; it traces, by means of its rays projected into the distance, a golden track which the logician has to follow to arrive at the port of his conclusion. Intuition and reasoning

---

[1] Schopenhauer, op. et t. cit., pp. 68, 69.

interpenetrate ; intuition makes the beginning, deduction carries on the work, but they are always in collaboration.

Nevertheless, the rôle of intuition differs from that of reasoning. Bergson deserves the credit for having best distinguished between them :—

" The intelligence treats everything mechanically ; instinct (that is to say intuition when it is conscious) proceeds, if we may thus speak, organically ; it does but continue the work by which life organizes matter. The intelligence is absorbed in the utilization of brute matter ; instinct remains within itself. Intelligence is turned towards inert matter, instinct towards life. Intelligence is the luminous kernel around which instinct, even when elevated to intuition only forms a vague nebulosity. Knowledge properly so called is reserved for pure intelligence ; intuition allows us to grasp what the fruit of intelligence cannot give us . . . By means of the sympathetic communication which it establishes between ourselves and all other living things, by the power which it has to enlarge our consciousness, it introduces us into the true domain of life, which is reciprocal interpenetration, indefinitely continued creation. Intelligence is adapted to matter and intuition to life. The reason why the consciousness is thus cloven into intuition and intelligence is that it needs to apply itself to matter at the same time as it follows the current of life. The essence of reasoning is to enclose us in the bounds of data ; thus positive science is the work of pure intelligence. But action, thanks to intuition, breaks the circle : the effort which we make to pass beyond pure understanding introduces us into something vaster where our understanding is cut off, and from which it has been obliged to detach itself." [1]

Although they are very distinct, intuition and intelligence interpenetrate : " Intelligence and instinct began by interpenetrating and have preserved something

---

[1] Bergson, op. cit., pp. 178–218.

of their origin. They are never pure; a fringe of intelligence always exists around instinct."[1]

Maine de Biran is less explicit on this point than Bergson, and sees in intuition a special, transitory, and more or less conscious form of knowledge : " It is not our common mode of knowledge. It comes at moments. It is accompanied by a certain effacement of consciousness." What does this mean ? Is intuition anything but instinct become conscious, as Bergson thinks ? It is a simple difference of degree. In intuition, there is synthetic or diffused consciousness ; in reasoning, the consciousness which is clear and distinct is rather analytical.

That is why Joseph de Maistre sees in this intuition the initial inspiration which seems independent of the work of dialectics, which it nevertheless sets going : " Genius does not move by leaning on syllogism. Its mien is free ; it is seen to arrive and no one has seen it on the way."[2]

It is also Caro's opinion : " It is this heart of science, this impulse of an act of faith, which in Kepler's case created astronomy ; which, with Colombus, saw the earth as a whole for the first time ; which created, in the case of Newton and Leibniz, the infinitesimal calculus. It is this which acts every day in every invention, in every conquest by the human mind, often without our being able to perceive the bond which unites the movement of the sciences to its mystical point of departure, to the initial impulse which drives it forward. Gratry calls this new form of science, this germ of all great inspirations, innate science."[3]

Finally, Paliard, summing up opinion on this matter, expounds in his turn a solution which, without being final, is to be kept in mind.

" The intuitionists reproach the dialecticians with substituting the artificial for the real, with abandoning

[1] Ibid.
[2] *Soirées de Saint Petersbourg*, ii, x^e entretien.
[3] Caro, *Philosophie et philosophes*, Paris, 1888, p. 228.

life, or with covering it thickly with a veil of logical conventions which are interposed between us and reality . . .

" The dialecticians reproach the intuitionists with reducing knowledge to fugitive impressions, more or less illusory and without attachment to anything stable . . .

" There is a point of view from which the philosophy of intuition and the philosophy of the concept are not incompatible. Our feeling for reality animates the whole reflective and constructive development of thought. On the other hand, the artificiality which is found in the concept is a necessity of nature . . .

" The conceptual milieu breaks and perhaps dissipates thought, but it is necessary ; it allows intuition to propagate itself. In short, intuition is always charged with some concepts, reflection is always illuminated by some intuition." [1]

On the whole, Paliard's thought meets that of Bergson : " Intuition charged with some concepts " recalls the fringes of intelligence which subsist around instinct.

These analyses are well founded, but in our view not sufficient to explain the whole mechanism of consciousness.

(d) Proposed Explanation

We have seen that the psychic force is divided between feeling, thought and activity. But there is reciprocal interpenetration of these three elements : all thought preserves an element of feeling and, in action, there is at once activity, feeling and thought.

All the same, these factors are not distributed in equal and constant proportions. These proportions are variable, and usually inverse : if the factor of feeling grows, the intellectual factor diminishes. This variation is true in general of all knowledge, and hence is also true for intuition and reasoning. Now we know that consciousness is more distinct in reasoning than in

[1] Paliard, Jacques, *Intuition et réflexion, Esquisse d'une dialectique de la connaissance*, Paris, 1925, pp. 160-2.

intuition derived from instinct. Thus intuition is a knowledge of which the intellectual factor is weak while the feeling factor is high. Reasoning, on the contrary, is knowledge which the feeling factor is weak while the representative factor is high. Intuition is above all a felt knowledge while reasoning is before all an intelligible knowledge, that is to say an explanatory knowledge.

These two processes of knowledge, which are different in their method, are also different in duration. In the case of intuition, divination occurs at the first glance at the reality, and we go to the heart of the object studied without the help of any intermediary. In reasoning, we advance step by step, depending upon known elements for our power to penetrate into the unknown. We may thus say that intuition is a direct, all-round, instantaneous grasp, a confused synthesis ; reasoning is a progressive statement : a slow, clear, and distinct analysis.

On the other hand, in a demonstration, intuition will give us the point of departure, since this is either undemonstrable or regarded as already demonstrated, and in either case an object of immediate knowledge. Intuition will also suggest, through affective tendencies, the point of arrival, the final conclusion, since reasoning, from the point of view of psychology, has no other value than that of precisifying and justifying this conclusion. Reasoning thus becomes the development of an intuition which plays the part of principle, and the justification of a second intuition which plays the part of conclusion. In short, the sum total of rational knowledge is a process of reasoning between two intuitions, an analysis between two syntheses.

V. IN ALL KNOWLEDGE, CONSCIOUS FACTORS AND UNCONSCIOUS FACTORS MAY BE DISTINGUISHED BY ANALYSIS

In this interpenetration of the various aspects of psychic force taken two by two, thought and feeling, feeling and activity, intuition and reasoning, we are now able to disentangle the conscious and the unconscious phases. Let us begin with sensibility.

(a) *In Sensibility*

In a general way, sensibility implies, if it is conscious, a certain degree of memory. Hence, every time that this memory fails, there will be unconsciousness in sensibility. " Consciousness," says Goblot, " might very well be a sensibility of the second degree. To be conscious is to feel that one is feeling . . . In order that my sensibility may become conscious, it is necessary that I should grasp, at each instance of my own existence, a little more than the absolute present of my subjective state ; it is necessary that, at each present instant, I should seize with my present state a little of my immediate past : it is necessary that this past be present. Consciousness cannot work without a certain degree of memory which is neither the recall nor the return of a memory picture, nor its conservation in a virtual form, but which is, properly speaking, and in spite of the strangeness of the terms, the persistence and hence the presence of the immediate past. Sensibility remains unconscious in so far as this memory fails." [1] If we further remark that this memory is impossible when sensibility falls below a certain degree, we discover an endless number of cases where sensibility remains unconscious because it has not sufficient tonality. We thus have in succession, unconsciousness and consciousness in sensibility, since there is variation in its intensity, and hence in memory.

We thus have to take into account, in estimating this consciousness and unconsciousness, the degrees of sensibility : " Every time," says Wundt, " that the possibility of a linkage of sense impressions is given us as a result of our physiological organization, consciousness will exist . . . The basis of the unity of consciousness

[1] Goblot (E.), *Le Système des sciences*, Paris, 1922, pp. 156–7.

is, in fact, the connection of the whole nervous system. Hence the domain of conscious life includes manifold degrees ; each degree is measured by the faculty of associating impressions."[1] Consciousness or unconsciousness will thus exist according as this linkage is or is not realized. Now it may be realized more or less ; all degrees are possible. By virtue of this gradation, which may be supposed infinite, there is an insensible passage from consciousness to unconsciousness. In short, says Wundt, " a positive decision on the matter of the non-existence of consciousness will never be possible."[2]

Wundt, however, admits the unconscious phase in sensibility, since he supposes it to be at the origin of feeling : " Feeling must always rest upon the process of unconscious conclusion by which the modification of our internal state, which is brought about by sensation or representation, is determined as being a subjective representation."[3] We thus find consciousness and unconsciousness in feeling. " Feeling," says Grote, " is the conscious product of the unconscious estimation of certain relationships." Thus, as Fouillée says, the intellectual operation which is the cause of feeling, is unconscious, while the feeling itself, resulting from this process, is conscious. Thus unconsciousness would be in the cause and consciousness in the effect.[4] But at what precise moment is this ascent from unconsciousness to consciousness in sensibility effected ? At the moment when the impression of effort appears : " All impressions which come from the organs," says Maine de Biran, " are not transformed into ideas with participation of consciousness. As obscure perceptions, they form the basis of the immediate feeling that we exist . . . Consciousness exists if we experience the impression of effort, which is a proper and original element of personal life, and if

---

[1] Wundt, *Psychologie physiologique*, p. 219.
[2] Op. cit., p. 224.
[3] Op. cit., p. 165.
[4] Fouillée, *Psych. des idées-forces*, ii, p. 99.

affections and intuitions are localized in some region of the resistant continuum formed by the locomotive system. But in that case we have attention : " We exert effort in order to arrange the motive organ so as to receive the impression better." Now when we are speaking of effort, we are speaking of constraint, opposition, contrary activity. The soul rises from unconsciousness to consciousness, says Bergson, " at the moment of its conflict with matter." [1]

To sum up, unconsciousness and consciousness succeed one another in sensibility. In unconsciousness, memory of the immediate past defaults, the linkage of sensorial impressions is impossible, feeling is in the state of incubation in the form of latent judgment, there is no effort, no localization of affective action, no attention. In consciousness, the immediate past persists in memory, the sensorial impressions are associated, feeling appears as the effect of unconscious work, we have effort, attention, and localization of sensorial impressions.

(b) *In Activity*

If we consider it as a whole, activity is the result of our whole past life : for we act for the most part according to our character, and this innate or acquired character appears to us, at the moment of action, as an indivisible domain, which has no doubt its conscious regions, but consists mainly of a vast unconscious territory. It is thus exactly true to say, following Bergson, " No doubt we only think with a small part of our past (we shall later add some reservations to this first statement) : but it is with our whole past, including our original cast of soul, that we desire, wish, act." [2] And since " the cerebral mechanism has forced almost the whole of it into the unconscious ", it is clear that these unconscious factors

---

[1] Biran, *Memoire sur les perceptions obscures* ; Paliard, *Le raisonnement selon M. de Biran*, p. 20.

[2] Bergson, *L'évolution créatrice*, p. 6.

have a very considerable place in our activity. On the other hand, " the cerebral mechanism only introduces into consciousness what serves a useful purpose." [1] The consciousness and the unconscious thus play their parts in activity : the latter the part of vague preparation for action ; the former the part of precise determination. Two cases are possible : either one action alone is possible, or several may be envisaged. In the first case there is no choice, hence no consciousness. In the second, preliminary deliberation is requisite, and hence, as decision implies knowledge, we have consciousness.

We thus have found the necessary place of unconsciousness and consciousness in the act itself. But let us go farther. Out of what does this act arise ? From a tendency a kind of predisposition to future action. Now we have seen that the active tendency, and a certain emotion serving to uphold it, always co-exist. One of two things happens : either " the tendency is immediately satisfied"; in this case the emotion, often unknown, which served as its invisible accompaniment, remains in the unconscious ; or " the tendency requires for its satisfaction a new adaptation " ; in this case a certain resistance is necessary, and consequently, according to the theories of Biran and Paulhan, the emotion is reinforced : the phenomenon becomes fully conscious. Thus, at the dawn of activity, in the tendencies which prepare for it, there is, according to circumstances, unconsciousness or consciousness [2]; unconscious, if the activity is immediate, consciousness, if the activity is retarded.

Up to the present, we have considered activity in its preparation, and in its relations with emotion. In truth, there is unconsciousness or consciousness, not in the activity itself, but in its emotive preparation. Let us now examine activity itself.

First of all, when a tendency is in conflict with a group of tendencies, and the act does not take place, the emotion is very lively. These inhibitory tendencies

[1] Ibid.   [2] Godfernaux, op. cit.

are often unconscious. Furthermore, Biran has shown us " those silent activities " at the basis of the organism, which change the direction of ideas : feeling of uneasiness, need of action, etc.[1]

Finally, in ordinary activity, we find arrest and return of consciousness. In fact, says Paulhan, " Consciousness is not produced when the psychic forces are not in some degree split up." [2] Thus, if one is absorbed by an occupation, the psychic forces preserve their unity, and consequently, consciousness of what one is doing is lost. But when an interruption comes, this dynamic aggregate is ruptured, and consciousness of what one is doing reappears.

Finally, therefore, activity is unconscious in its distant preparation, in its release when the given action is the sole possible, when it meets with no resistance, and when it is continuous. It is conscious, when the possible acts are manifold, when there is deliberation, retardation, or discontinuity.

(c) In Intuition

We may now consider the two forms of knowledge ; and first, intuition.

" It is almost always manifested in a sudden and unexpected fashion, often even at the moment when the scientist is beginning to doubt the possibility of finding the solution of his problem . . . It springs up unexpectedly under particularly favourable conditions. During a walk on the mountains, on the shores of a Swiss lake, wonderfully illuminated, or out at sea in brilliant moonlight, in general, in circumstances where the attention of the thinker is distracted from the problem which preoccupies him, and is in ecstasy before the beauties of Nature." [3]

[1] Biran, *Memoire sur les perceptions obscures, passim.*
[2] Paulhan, *Les phenomenes affectifs et les lois de leur apparition,* p. 53.
[3] Cyon, *Dieu et Science,* p. 192.

If intuition in itself is conscious, it has been immediately preceded by unconscious operations.

At what moment is this sudden illumination produced ? After long preparation : Newton established the law of universal attraction by always thinking about it. " Intuition is only given," says Pasteur, " to him who has undergone long preparation for receiving it." It is often in the morning on waking up that these intuitive ideas spring up : " One has the impression that the appearance of these ideas has been the cause of waking up. One seeks to establish a connection between the new idea and those with which the mind was preoccupied before sleep. This connecting chain appears slowly ; the links which preceded the apparition of the intuitive idea are missing. The greater part of these ideas would have remained unconscious or would only have reached consciousness in a fragmentary state." [1]

Around intuition, and in intuition itself, what is the field of consciousness, and what is that of the unconscious ? According to preceding analysis, the intellect supplies the data, it does not create. On the other hand, the intuition is the vision of the new thing, but this apperception is conscious. The unconscious thus occupies neither the intellectual zone which, long before the intuition, prepared it, nor the very brilliant luminous point which is the intuition itself, instinct become conscious. The unconscious occupies the region around the place where the intuition is to burst forth ; chronologically, it precedes the latter as smoke precedes fire.

So much as regards time. But what is the object which remains unconscious ? It is not the precise point contemplated in intuition, since this point is clearly perceived by the instinct become conscious, and is presented with a gesture which excludes uncertainty. Is it the rational antecedent, that is to say, the long study which prepared the way for the uprush of the intuition ? Impossible : these well directed investigations

[1] Cyon, op. cit., pp. 194, 195.

were known to the consciousness, since logical reasoning incited them. It is the bond which attaches the object of intuition to the object of previous investigations, a kind of invisible *nexus* which forms a bridge between the illuminated region of research and the brilliantly lit spot of the discovery.

But we can be still more exact. With Biran and Paliard we see an intuition in the conclusion of a chain of reasoning, an intuition which is a kind of luminous projection, and, " thanks to the intellectual memory which effects the synthesis of the successive steps, allows the whole chain of reasoning to be seen." [1] It is thus that after the painful ascent of a mountain, we take in at a single glance the whole range of the road we have traversed. Intuition thus becomes, according to Rignano's expression, " the vision of the validity of a general demonstration." [2] But in this case, what is unconscious is not the synthetic panorama, which is a direct object of intuition, and consequently perceived in its totality ; it is the detail, it is the particular thing noted when the phases of the reasoning were succeeding one another. It was conscious at the moment, but is no longer so when intuition in its sweep fixes its attention on the synthesis as a whole, neglecting the diversity of the parts.

(d) In the Stages of Rational Knowledge

Leaving the domain of intuition, it remains for us to find the position of consciousness and the unconscious in rational knowledge. This is a regular march towards a goal which is seen more or less clearly ; one might thus suppose, at first sight, that it is a pathway perpetually flooded with light, on which there is no room for the mysterious activity of the unconscious.

We have already seen, when studying the facts, that it is nothing of the kind. It is not merely in optics and

[1] Paliard, op. cit., p. 131,
[2] Rignano, op. cit., p. 170.

acoustics that interference modifies the key, of light or
of the waves of sound : these encounters, which result
in obscurity or greater brilliance, are found in the complex
phenomena of the most rational knowledge.

Let us follow the various stages of this process :
perception, recollection, association, intention, mental
selection, imaginative activity, formation of logical
connections, judgment and reasoning. Everywhere we
can distinguish an obscure fringe at the side of the region
illuminated by consciousness.

Let us commence with perception. It follows upon
sensation. Now, says Wundt, every time that, as a result
of our physiological organization, the possibility of a
linkage of sense impressions is given us, consciousness
will exist. The basis of the unity of consciousness is, in
fact, the connection of the whole nervous system.[1] Thus
whenever this linkage is either impossible or incomplete,
there is unconsciousness or attentuated consciousness.
Maine de Biran enlarges still further this domain of more
or less known perceptions. He includes affective
impressions of vision due to tone, shade, tint, without
perception properly so-called ; auditive perceptions
resulting from sound vibrations too weak to be perceived ;
silent activities changing the direction of ideas because,
without being known to us, they proceed from the depths
of the organism, etc. Besides, adds Biran, all degrees
are possible in this alternation between consciousness
and unconsciousness : " An unconscious act in its first
stage becomes perceptive and itself perceived. Others,
being too intense, benumb the faculty, whence the loss
of consciousness ; finally in our acts, the field of pure
impression, of perception, or consciousness, varies
unceasingly ; one region invades another or gives way
to it ; the consciousness of ourselves oscillates and
changes its position unceasingly." [2]

[1] Wundt, *Psychologie physiologique*, p. 219.
[2] Maine de Biran, *Mémoire sur les perceptions obscures*, pp. 11, 12,
13, 20.

But the concepts present to the mind have to be associated. Let A, B, C, D, E, F, be a certain number of these ideas. Why should A be bound to C and D rather to B and E or F ? The reason is that feeling has intervened. We shall thus have a clear notion of the result when once the connection has operated. But the point of departure of its mechanism has escaped us. The field of the unconscious in association is thus necessary very great.

A selection has, however, been necessary. Why are the materials of reasoning retained under a particular form ? To say that feeling has made one idea rather than another appear, is not to indicate the cause. Is not sensibility itself at the service of another idea ? We believe that it is stimulated by a more general idea, by a directing intention which enlists in its service the feelings and secondary ideas. This is the part of Rignano's opinion which we have to retain.[1] But attention is necessary to bring about this elimination and choice. Consequently the will plays its part in the elaboration of this association, but it is often unconscious and seemingly based on feeling ; one wills without thinking about it. Thus, in the mechanism of association there is unconsciousness, either at the point of departure, a general idea which is not thought about, or in the feeling which inspires the secondary ideas, or in the act of will, the spontaneous operation of which seems to be mistaken for mental selection, which, however, it directs.

Meanwhile, we do not think without images ; our associations are essentially the grouping of images. We must thus seek in the imagination, the power which creates these images, for the conscious and unconscious past. Fundamentally, we may, with Segond, regard it as " a power which creates the universe of images, the creative intuition of this universe ".[2] But in its potential state, its pure state, it escapes consciousness, " practically

[1] Rignano, op. cit., p. 93.
[2] Segond (J.), *L'imagination*, Paris, 1922, p. 18.

speaking, it is identifiable in the orientation of the images which it organizes ".

Let us consider it in its product, the image. This is a revival of the sensation and the perception, the sensation being weaker and the perception modified by individual feeling. It acts upon the senses, producing a tendency to movement, and causing the feeling which it expresses to be experienced. But consciousness grasps neither the mechanism of its formation nor the link which attaches it to a sensation and a movement. The consciousness has a clear notion of its apparition only.

Let us pass on to the combination of images brought about by creative imagination. This association is preceded by a dissociation, and governed by the law of interest, that is to say, by a feeling. In fact, as experience teaches us, the images are superposed in accordance with their resemblance to one another. The part common to these images is alone brought into relief. But this elimination of the differences is mechanical, never reflected upon, and hence always unconscious.

It may be said that the mind gives the first impulse and this is most often true. It then plays the part of determining the end in view, it orientates ; but the evocation of ideas and images, converging towards this end, remains spontaneous and more or less unconscious in its point of departure. What remains conscious is the vision of this procession of images once they have been associated, and not of their birth itself.[1]

Furthermore, there will be consciousness and unconsciousness in the discoveries suggested by the creative imagination. What is a discovery, if not " an unforeseen relation ", as Claude Bernard says ? But if it is unforeseen, it is not so, as a relation, at the moment when it is conceived : it is then conscious. It is unforeseen as regards the elements which prepare and constitute it. In other words, I know clearly the sense of A/B when this relation is given me. But I did not know beforehand

[1] Cf. Joly, L'imagination, passim ; Joyau, op. cit., passim.

the possibility of bringing A and B into relation : thus, previously to its appearance in consciousness, this relation was unconscious, since it could not spring out of nothing.

In fact, therefore, we meet the unconscious in imagination at three distinct moments : at the origin, in the faculty itself, in pure imagination ; then in the formation of the image and in its motive and sensitive properties ; finally in dissociations, which are the prelude to combinations, and in the evocation of secondary ideas. What is conscious is the directing idea and the vision of the result, of the artistic creation, the discovery, or the invention.

Let us now consider the logical relationships which constitute judgment and reasoning. The latter, since it is composed of linked judgments, is the same in origin as the former. The essential question to consider is thus the following : is not judgment essentially conscious ? Do we not make an unintelligible statement when we speak of unconscious judgment ?

Let us first of all note, with Ribot, " that our consciousness is temporal only and not spatial. We can thus know nothing in any but a successive form." According to the context he is dealing here with conscious knowledge. Our knowledge is thus a process which operates in time : the elements of our consciousness follow one another as moments of time follow one another. We must thus represent it either as a series of discontinuous points or as a continuous luminous trail. The choice must be made If we regard knowledge as a continuity of consciousness, we must also admit that there is a continuity of attention ; for, as we showed at the beginning of this study there is no consciousness without some degree of attention. Now everyone's experience proves that this continuity of attention never exists in fact, and remains impossible in principle. Rejecting this second alternative, we have to accept the first : knowledge is discontinuous. It remains logical, it implies elements which attract one another, which link up, but we see them in succession, and we do not even see them all. Logically, it is doubtless an uninterrupted chain, otherwise the necessary bond between cause and effect would be wanting : such knowledge would be illusory. But psychologically, we do not see and we cannot see all the links of the chain. Hence to those moments of absolute inattention or of diminished attention there correspond, in knowledge, inevitable breaks in continuity, that is to say, intervals of unconsciousness.

Let us now regard ideas as forces. If the idea is released, it acts of necessity. If two ideas are similar, they act by reinforcing one another ; if two ideas are contrary but unequal, the stronger realizes itself ; if finally the two ideas are equal and opposite, their action is neutralized. Let us note that, in the first and the fourth case, consciousness is only partial, since, if the action is necessary, it partly suppresses conscious reflection ; for, as Paulhan says, " to reflect is to experience the resistance of a new phenomenon aroused in the mind ". And here there is no new phenomenon and hence no resistance. On the other hand, when the action of the two equally powerful ideas is apparently cancelled, it exists none the less, but it is not seen. In every case, there was a moment when the force of the idea was not yet operative. It was in the potential state ; it existed, however, but in the unconscious state. In short, if we consider the dynamics of ideas, we distinguish in succession phases of unconsciousness and consciousness in a discontinuous progress.

But these ideas are about to be united by mental synthesis. In obedience to attractions which frequently remain unknown, they have to leave one system of associations in order to enter into another. This dissociation and reassociation are thus partially unconscious. But association does not necessarily imply junction ; the juxtaposition of two ideas is one thing, their fusion another. The latter, which is an essential element of mental synthesis, is an assimilation. Now we have no more knowledge of the motives serving as the point of departure for this logical junction, than we have of physiological assimilation. We only see the result, and we recognize that the result is legitimate. But the operation itself has escaped us. Thus in the mental synthesis which is the condition of all judgment, the assimilative operation is unconscious, and the result alone conscious.

Let us now examine the operation of the judgment. It is not simple, and analysis distinguishes three moments, all of which are necessary for the judgment to have psychological existence and logical value.

(*a*) First moment : The assertion of the person judging. " I think that . . ." is understood in every judgment ; it is the commencement of action, as Kant recognized. But it is clear that this proposition is not explicitly formulated by the consciousness.

(*b*) Second moment : I affirm that there is agreement between my thought and reality. If I say " Socrates is a wise man " I think that I am expressing a truth. This proposition is clearly conceived by the mind.

(*c*) Third moment : We affirm that what appears true to us has universal application : it is true for the whole world and for all time. But this modality of the thought has not been explicitly formulated. It remains unconscious.

Hence the second alone of these three assertions remains conscious. But is it necessarily so ? In common with Paulhan, we do not think so. " Consciousness," he says, " is not an essential element of the phenomenon. The play takes place, it is not necessary that it should be revealed. Internal perception causes us to recognize a phenomenon, it does not constitute it ; it is a second phenomenon grafted on the first, a second synthesis superposed on the first. But it does not give it its existence. Thus unconscious judgments are possible. The greater part of our judgments are unconscious. We

R

neglect one quality for another in harmony with our feelings.[1]

All the same, when presented in this form, Paulhan's opinion implies a contradiction. He distinguishes between a first phenomenon which is not perceived, and a second phenomenon, that of consciousness, which is perceived. But is a phenomenon which is not perceived a phenomenon ? Every phenomenon reveals a fact or a state. This phenomenon, as far as it is one, is, thus necessarily perceived, necessarily conscious, otherwise we are ceasing to speak clearly. But what can exist without being revealed is the psychical fact or state. We can thus distinguish the psychical fact or state from its conscious manifestation. The contradiction disappears.

But are we then obliged to admit the epiphenomenon theory of consciousness ? Not at all. If consciousness exists, it is the consciousness of a mental state. It is not an empty consciousness, which would be without meaning. Thus when mental facts are said to be conscious, no distinction is made between the facts and their internal perception. But there is co-existence of the facts and of the consciousness of the facts.

But these facts or these states of mind can exist without being revealed. Their existence does not necessarily bring with it their internal manifestation in conscious form. Thus we no longer have unconscious phenomena, but unconscious facts, and, if we speak of phenomena, they are necessarily conscious.

If the judgment can be an unconscious state or fact, how is that brought about which is the essential of judgment, namely, the connection between subject and attribute ? The affirmation or negation of this relationship are conscious acts. But to affirm or to deny is to state a perceived agreement or disagreement. The apperception of this agreement or disagreement is also a fact of consciousness. But one only perceives what

[1] Paulhan, *L'activité mentale et les éléments de l'esprit*, Paris, 1889, p. 122.

already exists, what is already present in the mind, and this object or present state is logically anterior to the act of mind which perceives it. In short, the existence of this object or of this state is anterior to its apperception. But, before this apperception, it is unconscious. There is thus, in every judgment, a moment of unconsciousness. And this moment is necessary. It is impossible, in fact, for the consciousness to perceive what is not already in the mind in some fashion. But how can the object be thus present in the mind without being seen ? By the "impressed element" of Aristotle and the Scholastics, a kind of imprint is produced in the senses by the object and submitted to by the mind. That is one explanation. Another is as follows. The external object produces sensations in us ; by virtue of the principles of causality and substance, we interpret them by a process of reasoning which is not conscious : this is the theory of inference. Here the unconscious element is an instinctive interpretation of conscious sensation. In the two theories, a state of mind, an unconscious modification of the mind, has necessarily preceded the assertion of agreement or disagreement.

It may be agreed that this is true with reference to the judgment of perception. Is it so of all judgments ? Absolutely : for judging is affirming the relationship between two ideas presented to the mind ; that is to say, manifesting a state or modification of the mind in relationship to these ideas. Now this modification or this state cannot be revealed unless it logically precedes this revelation. That is to say, at a given moment they constitute an unconscious mental state. At the last analysis we always find an unconscious phase in judgment.

It may be said that these are useless subtilties. If I affirm a relationship, it is because I see it : thus my act is conscious. That is understood, but you cannot see what is not there. Do you say that it is the act of seeing itself which creates the relationship ? But what relationship ? The relationship between A and B ? The fact is that the concepts A and B exist prior to your affirmation, and further are such, in the nature of their being, that they can be put into relationship. In any case, A and B and the mental state created by their co-existence in the mind must be imagined as previous to any assertion concerning their relationship. Thus an obscure phase necessarily precedes the conscious affirmation.

The foregoing argument is *a priori*. Let us consider whether the facts confirm the analysis. Let us take everyday judgments, such as we express at a given moment concerning men and things. When am I able to say of my neighbour, for example, that he is a " good fellow " ? When I have had a sufficiently long experience of him, after facts have produced an impression upon me, without my having been preoccupied with the judgment which I was eventually to make. This judgment is thus the revelation of a mental state which was formed without my knowledge, and of which only the last stage has been grasped by consciousness. At the end of my literary studies, I may thus sum up my opinion of Voltaire : Voltaire had a very lucid intelligence, but an evil heart. How has this double attribution been brought about in me ? How has this double judgment been formulated ? When I express it, I am clearly aware that it translates my thought. But can I know in an exact fashion how my thought has been elaborated ? Doubtless, by psychological analysis, I shall find the origin of my opinion in a series of readings which I have made of this author's works, or in a certain number of criticisms which I have heard ; perhaps also I must add to this my personal reflections. Thus, in a certain number of circumstances I was conscious of elements which were one day to serve for the production of my whole judgment concerning this writer. But in each of these circumstances, I was not thinking of this final expression of my thought. If I one day emit this judgment it is the reflection of an internal state which has been formed within me, without the clear concurrence of my consciousness.

My judgment, which is conscious in its translation, was unconscious in its elaboration. It is unnecessary to analyse other opinions. Judgments on an historical personage, new convictions which suddenly burst forth in the soul of a convert, bold assertions thrown into a discussion without their having been foreseen at the outset of the dialectical game—all these are facts which corroborate our theory. The affirmation of the judgment is like the manifestation of a mental crystallization which has been formed in obscurity ; we are conscious of the appearance of the crystal, but we have not been present or presided at its formation. To sum up, the operation of the judgment is unconscious as regards the mental modification which elaborates it, and conscious as regards the proposition which expresses the result of it.

We may now pass to reasoning which is a series of judgments linked one to another. The question before us is this : are all the links of this chain necessarily conscious ? If some are so, and others are not in certain cases, which are those which are conscious and which are those which cannot be so ?

In order to make this distinction, we must first consider what is the essential nature of reasoning. Spencer calls it " a classification of relationships ". This definition is exact, but it does not teach us anything concerning the mechanism of classification. For in order to classify, we must have a conducting thread. We therefore prefer to say with Binet that " reasoning is the transition from a known fact to an unknown fact by way of a resemblance ".[1] It is in fact by virtue of this similitude that two images unite by their common points. But is it necessary that this associative force, in order to be efficacious, should be notified to the consciousness ? In no way, for if the image is formed without our knowledge in imaginative work, why could it not fuse with others without our mind receiving warning ? " Two images follow one another in the mind," says Binet, " it

[1] Binet, *Psychologie du raisonnement*, p. 95.

matters little or no whether we are aware of their resemblance to one another, being similar, they set a common cellular element vibrating. This identity of seat produces all the results produced by a resemblance which is recognized and judged by conscious comparison." [1]

Thus, as Taine puts it, our mind has become "a polyp of images ". They are associated by resemblance in their origin, and are soon associated by contiguity. We thus find accomplished in all reasoning what is verified in external perceptions. Being born from the contact with objects, " the images form a whole which corresponds to the notion of a single object." Now we had no consciousness of their origin, which is the modification of the sensorial centres of the brain. Since the new images modify the old ones, we are equally ignorant of the new state which they create. A whole series of imaginative metamorphoses is effected without our knowledge. That is how it happens that the premises are unconscious in the majority of cases of reasoning. The conclusion alone, in many cases, is known. It appears to us as an isolated thought, because we have not noticed its obscure origins. In reality, the more or less original thought which enters consciousness is the last link of a chain. A thorough analysis of its content would reveal its points of attachment to the mental past. But when is this analysis made ? After the act, by virtue of the patient work of reflection. Hence at this moment, the reasoning is already finished.

Our critical study of the judgment explains this result. Reasoning is a chain of judgments linked together with a view to a conclusion which is to be justified. Hence, *a priori*, we can detect in each of these judgments the phase of unconsciousness which our preceding examination allows us to discover there. If all these judgments were presented under their regular form, as is alone the proposition which expresses the result,

[1] Op. cit., p. 116.

which is truly conscious, we should have in the ordinary syllogism an alternation between unconscious and conscious phases in the following manner :—

Major : Unconscious preparation, conscious expression,

Minor : Unconscious preparation, conscious expression.

Conclusion : Unconscious elaboration, conscious expression.

If we represent by a full line the conscious period and by a dotted line the unconscious period, we obtain the following scheme of discontinuity :—

Unconscious. <u>Conscious.</u> Unconscious. <u>Conscious.</u>
....
<u>Major.</u>   <u>Minor.</u>

Unconscious. <u>Conscious.</u>
....
<u>Conclusion.</u>

But in this hypothesis, we have supposed that all the results of successive judgments have been revealed to consciousness. In the majority of cases the mind only has knowledge of the last judgment, of the conclusion. All that has preceded it and prepared for it, the successive images which have modified one another by invisible reactions, have remained in shadow as far as consciousness is concerned. The whole reasoning is then presented in the form of a judgment, the mute elaboration of which has been prolonged, and the result of which is notified to consciousness in the form of a sudden flash. The scheme representing this mysterious evolution is then a dotted line ending in a full line.

Preparation.

Unconscious Major. Unconscious Minor.   <u>Revelation.</u>
....
<u>Conclusion.</u>

If we refer to our long inquiry concerning the unexpected manner in which fruitful ideas have been revealed to inventors, we shall easily understand the character of this sudden vision of truth. In appearance it is an intuition. In reality, it is the outcome of long deductions the materials of which have been consciously introduced into the mind, while their mysterious combination has escaped logical reason. The final conclusion alone penetrates into consciousness in the form of a sudden revelation.

Here is our conclusion. Not only may reasoning be unconscious, but it frequently is so. In this case the consciousness only grasps the manifest results of the various judgments, sometimes only the final conclusions. All the other modifications of the mind, and the fusions or reductions of images, have remained unconscious.

VI. The Place and the Relative Importance of Feeling, Intuition, Reasoning, Activity, Consciousness and Unconsciousness in all Intellectual Construction

We may now make an end to our long analysis. It was necessary to allow us to grasp in the minutest details the part played by the various factors. It must be completed by a synthesis which it has rendered possible, the synthesis of these various elements in intellectual construction. We must distinguish the preparation of the creative work, the conception of the directing idea, the modification of this hypothesis, and the verification of its final expression.

1. *Preparation*

First of all, has this word any independent meaning, any significance in itself, apart from the hypothesis ? Absolutely none. If I prepare myself, it is for something : I have a motive for my activity a preformed orientation. But what is this ? I have not yet made a choice. No exact idea is directing my researches. Whether I am called Newton, Ampère, Renan, or Berthelot, I make observations, I apply myself to special study. I evidently do not do this without an object, since the sequence of my thought appears coherent. Meanwhile, I cannot yet say to myself that I am doing it for the purpose of establishing a certain law or building a certain machine.

Why then does this general orientation exist ? What is the origin of this taste of Pasteur for crystals, the passion of Cuvier for animal or vegetable remains, the fascination exercised by geometrical figures on mathematicians when still children ? Either from atavism, or from a personal aptitude antecedent to all experience. In both cases, the future scientist has been guided by nature. Strange as this expression appears, the first direction of his mind was unconscious.

By virtue of this original impulse, his mind enjoys making observations which harmonize with its tastes. These bear fruit in sensation and feeling, and hence emotive states, at least partially conscious. However, without always thinking about it, he benefits by lessons received, new facts learned, communications received from seekers like himself ; and thus his sensibility, his intelligence, and his activity are incessantly modified, and create in him a new personality, rich in all the acquisitions of the past, and full of unsuspected possibilities.

Little by little, he becomes conscious of it ; he sees what others have done, he foresees what remains to be done. Under the influence of feeling, the images of what he has already seen combine and organize themselves within him ; a new image appears ; it is the hypothesis, the analogy, the directing idea.

2. *The Conception of the Directing Idea*

It is a surprise, for the new arrival was not expected in this form : its original character was not prepared for. The mind, however, recognizes its own product ; on reflection, it sees its most cherished ideas ; consequently in this intuition of something new, there is a kind of

recognition of the past. But this survival of the past
in the new concept is first unconscious; critical
examination by the mind discovers it after the event.
On the contrary, the character of novelty is immediately
perceived by the consciousness.

3. The Modifications of the Hypothesis

The directing idea is born. But only experience can
show whether it is able to survive. We now have, as the
experimental process unfolds, a whole series of sensations,
imaginative constructions, and reasonings, for the
purpose of determining the result of the experiments :
We have thus a series of feelings and images, of operations
which are at one time conscious and at other times
unconscious. But as the facts do not sufficiently confirm
the preconceived theory, this hypothesis has to be
modified to some extent.

Others besides Pasteur, Darwin, and Claude Bernard
have been brought by the lesson of experience to re-model
a system of ideas. All those who, as editors of reviews
or authors of books are accustomed to literary invention,
know that they are often obliged to modify their plans
for articles or the arrangement of their theme because
their directing idea has been found to conflict with the
facts. Hence those numerous attempts and successive
retouchings which the theory in process of formation
undergoes. Finally, a halt is made at its last expression.
How has this ultimate crystallization been formed ? It
was, as it were, presaged in the course of the examination
of its predecessors, and hence sensibility has played its
part in the matter ; it is revealed under the form of an
image, and hence it is the product of the imagination :
it flashes out suddenly with the unexpected brilliance of
an intuition, and nevertheless its modifications have been
introduced by processes of reasoning, unconscious of the
end towards which they were tending, but conscious of

each progressive step which they accomplished. We thus discover in the devious progress of its variations the fugitive trace of all psychical factors, sensible or intellectual, conscious or unconscious.

4. *Final Verification*

When the plan is formed, and the system settled on its main lines, the task of submitting it to the control of reason remains. In this work it is supported by feeling, the intense joy caused by the discovery, or an agonizing restlessness as the result of the difficult problems which are raised. The logic which directs the verification has an element of the unconscious in it, but most often the process is conscious; there is feeling at the base of the researches, but in general the work of verification is one of rational control.

In short, sensibility and intelligence, intuition and deduction, analysis and synthesis, unconsciousness and consciousness follow one another, interweave with one another, and interpenetrate in the actual mechanism of integral knowledge.

Conclusion

We have thus seen the process of integral knowledge as a whole. We have shown the solidarity of feeling, of thought, and of action. We have seen the regular succession and sometimes the interpenetration of unconscious and conscious elements in the work of knowledge. Knowing, in the full sense of the word, is not only perceiving a certain relation here and now; it is rather gathering in the present the harvest of the mental past; it is benefiting, in the conscious revelation of a law, by all the mysterious work which prepared for its incubation during many years. Knowing is doubtless perceiving in a flash of intuition a new relation, a fertile hypothesis, a splendid analogy; but it is above all associating the work of the past with the new idea by bonds in which sensibility has a place as well as reason, bonds formed by the creative imagination, at times in the mystery of unconscious life, at other times in the clear light of logic. To know fully is to have loved truth, it is to have sought for it passionately, and it is to have contributed to its discovery, under the influence of this ardent desire, all the powers of one's soul. In this sense, one cannot subscribe to Bergson's assertion : " We do not think with more than a small part of our past, but it is with our whole past, including our original cast of mind, that we desire, will, act." Why make this distinction ? If desire, will, and action appear now in a determinate manner as the result of our whole past life, why should the case be otherwise with our thought, since it contains an element of feeling, and also depends upon the will by way of the attention, and since in an unconscious form, our original cast of mind, our sensibility, and our activity have been prepared in the whole of our past ?

The unconscious is found as the mysterious agent of mental transformation in all phases of knowledge. It remains for us to consider under what form it operates ; whether, in the laboratory of the human mind, it is only an automatic recorder or a transformer of movements already begun. We require to know whether it is purely mechanical or whether at the same time it is dynamic. It would appear to be both in so far as it becomes æsthetic, that is to say, acts upon sensibility. These problems must be solved in order to enable us to apply the results obtained in the study of integral knowledge. For inventing is, in the first place, knowing, and hence performing a work of science ; in the second place, it is realizing something, and hence performing a work of art. And because, in the scientific field, knowledge is the essential objective, while the application of knowledge are rather a matter for industry, it will be a matter for us to consider above all the rational and the methodical aspect of scientific knowledge. Scientific invention is a superior theoretical knowledge. Hence the

unconscious, which we have found among the factors
of all knowledge, should logically have a place in the
long and patient elaboration of new systems, of fertile
theories, or of powerful machines. We propose to follow
it out by examining in turn its automatic aspect, its
dynamic form, and its æsthetic character.

Chapter II

THE RÔLE AND INSUFFICIENCY OF THE AUTOMATIC UNCONSCIOUS

Nature of the automatic unconscious—Its production—The rôle of the automatic unconscious—Insufficiency of the automatic unconscious—Conclusion : necessity for a dynamic unconscious.

WE shall have to find the extent of the automatic unconscious in scientific invention if, after having examined its nature, we consider the various ways in which it is produced, if we determine its rôle in the various mental operations, and if we find the reason for its insufficiency.

I. THE NATURE OF THE AUTOMATIC UNCONSCIOUS

This term is used to denote subconscious acts. These are " acts having the character of psychical acts, but escaping, at the moment they are effected, the consciousness ".[1] More precisely, " it is a psychological activity more or less unconscious in itself, but conscious in its point of departure and in its point of arrival, as well as by its projection into clear consciousness." [2] It is thus an intermittent unconscious, a succession of psychical states at one time conscious at another unconscious. Usually they are conscious at the moment of their full realization. In the case of the inventor or the scientist, an original idea strikes him. The mind ceases to think about it, but the idea is transformed without his knowledge ; one day it reappears in his consciousness completely modified, and associated with other ideas forming a group. The invention is realized.

[1] Dwelshauvers, *L'inconscient*, p. 34.
[2] Lahr, *Cours de philosophie*, Paris, 1926, vol. i, p. 62.

254

All the same, it is not a matter of purely mechanical activity. The soul is not an apparatus moved by an internal spring which imitates spontaneity and life. Nor is it a physiological automatism : the soul has an internal life which is not comparable to the release of a reflex in the spinal cord. It is a matter of psychological activity : a phenomenon, in origin psychological, works itself out beyond the zones of reflection and will ; at this moment it is no longer psychological, it is psychical. It then rises again into the domain of consciousness and thus becomes psychological again.

II. ITS PRODUCTION

We find it first of all in habits in general : The unconscious movements of the hand which are facilitated by haschisch, table turning, automatic writing, and table rapping, come from unconscious muscular tension.[1]

Pierre Janet has shown us the various manifestations of it in psychological automatism. In passion, it causes a procession of vague images to pass through our mind and drives us to act in harmony with these representations ; as a result of the association of ideas the appearance of one idea causes the idea which resembles it to rise up. Automatism also presides at the formation of images ; their simple association often takes the place of reasoning.[2]

We do not need to insist on the rôle of this unconscious in pathological states : catalepsy, somnambulism, and hypnotic suggestions. We may also remark that suggestion may be normal. The scientist who gives himself a certain idea by studying meditation is exercising auto-suggestion ; his idea will realize itself one day or another under one or another form.

In all these cases, as Herzen says, " an idea which disappears from consciousness does not thereby cease to

---

[1] Dwelshauvers, op. cit., pp. 34–112.
[2] Janet (Pierre), *L'automatisme psychologique, passim.*

exist ; it can continue to act in the latent state and, so to speak, below the horizon of consciousness. . . . In this subconscious state it may still have motor effects and influence on other ideas." [1]

In all cases we are dealing with " acts having all the characters of psychological acts excepting one : they are unknown to the subject. In that case, either the individual is unconscious of any act, or he is conscious of all acts excepting the one which he executes without being aware of it ".[2]

Dwelshauvers has recently experimented at Barcelona on the manner in which the unconscious acts in the production of a stimulated mental image :—

" In our sensations, as in our feelings, analysis proves the retention of events which act upon conscious life without, however, proceeding from it . . .".

A word is spoken aloud and the subjects of the experiment are asked to write down the image suggested by it.

When the stimulus word has been pronounced, the corresponding image is immediately produced. Sometimes it has various forms. Thus the word *tree* suggested two visual images, five particular images, of which two were of a cherry tree. Often an unconscious association is produced with another idea : For example, the word *eternity* awakens the idea of *God*.

If a whole thought is suggested, the images are stimulated by a word, but not by the whole proposition expressed. Furthermore, certain words are more suggestive than others : these are words expressing value.

In a general way, the visual image is more stable than the auditive image.

Representation is effected more easily when it is spontaneous than when an effort is made. Of thirty-one questions given to the experimental subjects, twenty-nine were affirmative. Reflection is thus injurious to the

---

[1] Quoted by P. Janet in *État mental des hystériques*, pp. 51, 52.
[2] Janet, *L'automatisme*, p. 225.

formation of images : the " polyp of images ", of which Taine speaks, grows, not in consciousness, but in the depths of the unconscious. That is why the production of representative images is so brilliant in the dream and in reverie ; the subconscious has free rein.

However, if the will does not favour the production of the image, it most frequently ensures its stability. Let us make a note of this point. The proverbial tenacity of scientists has maintained the continuity of their researches by keeping a directive scheme of the hypothesis before their imagination.[1]

Dwelshauvers showed the rôle of the unconscious in the formation of images. Abramowski makes a clear distinction between the image and the recollection, and by numerous experiments, shows how what is forgotten is preserved in the normal subconsciousness.

First of all, the image differs from the recollection as the part differs from the whole ; " the image is only a detail of the recollection ; the essential part of the recollection is its non-representative side, which is the most difficult to preserve by introspection. In a sense, one may even say that it is unconscious. Consequently, the recollection is an affective phenomenon partly intellectualized as an image. What then is recognition ? The perception of an object in its non-intellectual aspect, an affective phenomenon, a feeling of familiarity incorporated with the impression." [2]

But every perception itself contains two elements : one the pure impression, the second the intellectual elaboration by the attention.

" If the impression is received without attention, it is an intellectual psychical state. The perception is reduced to the state of a certain kind of *feeling*. When it is reduced to this state, the perception is the subconscious element inaccessible to thought, but influencing thought. . . ."

---

[1] Dwelshauvers, *Les Mecanismes subconscients*, pp. 2–41.
[2] Abramowski, *Le subconscient normal*, pp. 23–4.

" When the perception passes into forgetfulness, it produces for the latter a similar emotional reduction. That which is forgotten is preserved, not only physiologically, as a corresponding residual modification of the brain, but also psychically as a subconscious record, as an emotional equivalent of the past perception."

" It follows from this that, in the psychical world, nothing perishes, and that the whole past of the individual, the whole mass of what is forgotten and reproduced only partially and from time to time in conscious recollection, exists as a whole and constantly, as the equivalent of an enormous subconscious memory, which is uniform not differentiated by thought, and in the form of the emotional reduction of the past. Every moment lived through leaves behind its emotional equivalent, a trace, preserved in the subconscious, of its past existence.[1] "

The following are the conclusions of this author respecting the many forms under which the subconscious is produced :—

(1) The normal subconscious is intellectualized more easily than the morbid.

(2) The greater part of what is forgotten is only partially intellectualized. Recollections are thus more affective than representative.

(3) Other recollections are intellectualized in an indirect manner. These are facts which cannot be recalled but which are recognized when repetition occurs.

(4) The deepest layer of the forgotten, which is entirely lost to consciousness, is only revealed in affective states.

(5) Impressions received in a state of distraction form thoughts which are sketchy and unfinished. We then often have the production of the phenomenon known as paramnesia, or false memory, the feeling of having already seen or experienced something. An actual perception seems to be a memory, either because it really resembles an impression, or most often because under these conditions, the object is perceived in two

[1] Op. cit., pp. 136–7.

states : in a state of inattention and in a state of attention. In this second state, we have the impression of having seen the thing already because, an instant before, perception actually took place without being fully remarked. At the moment when full consciousness occurs, we thus have the idea of the "already seen". This is not a complete illusion : it is merely the recognition in full clarity of consciousness of the immediate past, which was recorded without full consciousness.

III. The Rôle of the Automatic Unconscious

Whatever its degree of obscurity, automatism exerts an influence which is easy to point out and to delimit, whether it is considered first of all in the series of intellectual operations, or whether it is seen in the special procedures which lead to discoveries and scientific inventions.

(a) It is a reproductive and non-deliberative power. Consequently, it may be looked upon as a reservoir which preserves syntheses previously constructed. But it is also a kind of regulator which causes stored-up elements to appear exactly in the order in which they were recorded. This is of great importance with regard to invention ; for the logical unconscious will unfold itself in the same manner as conscious dialectic.

This reservoir feeds all intellectual operations ; perception borrows from it in order to assume the special or individual colour which characterizes the latent judgment which is contained in perception ; the memory finds in it the materials for its recollections. For, in alliance with association of ideas, it receives from the latter bundles of impressions already built up, in such a fashion that the order of the reappearance of the forgotten is the same order which presided over its registration in the association. By virtue of these available elements, the imagination reconstructs after having dissociated, like a house-breaker of genius who raises the columns of a new temple upon the ruins which he has laid in heaps. By virtue of this mysterious provision of ideas, the orator and the philosopher form their deductions out of sight and without effort, finding within their reach the conclusive fact or the decisive argument. What would Descartes or Kant have done without these invaluable mental docks ? In order to criticize the systems of one's predecessors, it is necessary to know them and thus be able to bring into clear consciousness the hidden scroll of unconscious notions.

It is for this reason that all inventors have built up in their minds a rich capital of latent memories, which they have added to unknown to themselves, in proportion to their observations, reading, and experience, while awaiting the hour for their profitable utilization. All their intellectual habits, reinforced by the number, duration, and intensity of past acts and the comparison of their experiences, have predisposed them to their future conquest by making them heirs of their own mental past.

This explains for us the passion with which they amassed knowledge upon knowledge. Pascal worked for nine years at his calculating machine, a time full of observations which were noted and then forgotten, but stored in the unconscious. Leibniz acquainted himself with the works of Pascal, Fermat, and Cavalieri, before constructing his infinitesimal calculus ; he thus preserved, in the reservoir of his subconscious, the materials of which he was one day to make use. After having propounded the theory of the latent conservation of ideas, afterwards to be realized by memory, Laplace made use of this unconscious mechanism and pressed into his service notions borrowed from Buffon, and perhaps Kant, for the construction of his cosmic hypothesis. Ampère was enabled to publish his *Considerations on the Mathematical Theory of Games of Chance* by seven years of researches. The same work put to reserve was observed in the case of Gauss and Sully-Prudhomme before the discovery of their solutions. Finally, Henri Poincaré assembled the observations of fifteen years before deducing from them the fuchsian functions. In all these cases there were many breaks in the research, but each new acquisition played the part of a preparation for that following it.

We have seen that similar considerations apply to all the fields of invention—physical, biological, moral, and technical—which we have investigated in detail in this work; we may say that, using the word in its economic sense, the automatic unconscious forms the *capital* of genius.

But there are two ways in which capital may be utilized. For some it is simply a source of revenue, for others, better advised, it is an instrument of production, not in itself, but through the intermediary of labour. Wealth in gold or scrip would be sterile were it not fertilized by industry. All the same, the psychical wealth accumulated in the automatic unconscious would not itself suffice to produce anything new. We may now consider the reason for this fundamental impotence of the automatic unconscious, when left to itself, to bring forth scientific inventions.

IV. INSUFFICIENCY OF THE AUTOMATIC UNCONSCIOUS

Inventions are produced by the conjunction of creative imagination, of judgment, of reasoning, and above all of intuitive reasoning. They are rendered possible by memory, association, reproductive imagination, and habit.

Now it is easy to show that the automatic unconscious intervenes in the mechanism of the association of memory images, of the reproduction of images, and of the formation of habits. But no creation could be expected from the mere accumulation of facts which can be recalled and from a collection of images which can be made to reappear. Conservation is not development. The evocation of the past can only bring it back in the form in which it was buried ; and this does not enrich or enlarge it.

The work of improvement and true progress requires the intervention of intellectual faculties which alone are truly productive, reflective, and deliberative. The mind cannot use its reserves without the intervention of conscious reasoning.

First of all, the creative imagination makes use of associations in its combination, but under the control of reasoning. Genius cannot exist without the power of synthesis. Now, if the mental image is formed in spite of ourselves, the elements of which it is composed have always been perceived in the full light of logic previously to the invention taking place. On the other hand, the image is not simply the sum of the images composing it ; it is a new image. It has made use of pre-existing elements in its formation, and hence analysis can detect in it the traces of the materials so used. Now the essence of the invention will consist precisely in a new attribute, or a new relationship. The discovery of this cohesive power necessitates our going beyond the range of the automatic unconscious.

Might it not be in the domain of intuitive reasoning that these reserves of latent memories are called upon to fructify ? But how is this mysterious production to be conceived ? If it is true that the fertile idea is revealed by an intuition, it is not less certain that this light, shining in the night of unconscious incubation, is nothing but the external manifestation of an internal activity. Now the hypothesis thus revealed is a novelty, a creation, and has not been produced from the automatic store-house in its finished state. A store-house can only furnish us with elements which have been deposited in it. A clever idea which proceeded merely from automatism could not have anything original in it. It might be a composite idea, a kind of psychical resultant of previous ideas. But it could not constitute an invention.

It may be said that the automatic unconscious translates

the idea into movements and acts ; it thus finishes the idea. Is not this a kind of creation ? In the same way might not automatism effect the same development in the case of scientists and inventors ?

It is easy to see that we are not dealing with a case of real originality. If, as we have pointed out, every idea is linked with a movement this movement forming part of the idea and translating it externally, must not be confounded with the mental operation of genius which constructs a new system. In the elaboration of this there is a force added to automatic activity, and that is why this super production is an extraordinary fact, while the mechanisms linked with unreflecting activity form the course of our ordinary life.

V. CONCLUSION

The automatic unconscious is thus at the same time both necessary and insufficient. It nourishes genius with recollections and regulates their appearance, it furnishes the matter by which the imagination profits. It furnishes the mind with latent associations, the material of which is utilized by judgment and reasoning.

In order to render this reserve capital productive, in order to fertilize the creative imagination, to stimulate the reason, and give wings to genius, it is necessary, as we shall show, to pass beyond the region of pure automatism, and to take into consideration the latest energy of a dynamic unconscious.

CHAPTER III

THE NECESSITY FOR THE DYNAMIC UNCONSCIOUS IN INVENTION

Definition of the dynamic unconscious—It is a suggestion—
The dynamic unconscious effects the association of ideas—
It produces the productive work of the creative
imagination—The synthetic unconscious—Summary and
conclusion.

I. DEFINITION OF THE DYNAMIC UNCONSCIOUS

In a general way, we must understand by this term
" all the forms of unconscious activity, which, at a given
moment and in the normal state, influence our
mentality ".[1]

We are no longer dealing with those motor mechanisms
which blindly obey a mental synthesis pre-existing in
consciousness. We thus eliminate all those pathological
states which were already set aside in the case of automatism, whose possible influence is morbid, in no way
rational, and hence incapable of the creations of genius.

The question is thus reduced to the examination of
those ideas which are first of all repressed by consciousness,
and then, later, react secretly in the form of tendencies ;
of that reverie in which the most various images succeed
one another, often in an incoherent manner, but which,
one day, unexpectedly produces an original thought.
We have further to examine ideas first associated in
full consciousness, then forgotten, finally returning to the
threshold of consciousness in a daring form. We must
consider the many combinations effected by the silent
artistry of the imagination without any warning being
given to the logical reason of the transformation ; the
invisible upthrusts effected by the power of previous

[1] Dwelshauvers, *L'inconscient*, p. 112.

judgments ; conclusions forgotten for the moment, which later burst upon the consciousness under the brilliant form of an inspiration ; and finally, those enlargements of thoughts which, originating in the penumbra of a reverie, suddenly lay hold of the attention and result in profound meditation.

Finally, the dynamic unconscious expresses all the hidden influences, which have modified, which are modifying, and which will modify in the future, our psychical state. One word expresses all the shades of this activity : the word *suggestion*.

II. THE DYNAMIC UNCONSCIOUS IS, BEFORE ALL THINGS, A SUGGESTION

Let us first of all define the sense of this word, the significance of which has in our day been so extended as to become entirely vague.

" It is the effects of suggestion," writes Wundt, " which are the only states of consciousness aroused in us strong enough to resist—at least momentarily—contrary states of consciousness which tend to destroy them."

This is an exact definition, but it does not indicate one important character of the suggestion, namely, ignorance of the belief thus formed. On the other hand, Guyau is no more explicit in defining this mental operation as " the introduction of a practical belief which realizes itself ".[1] What is this, in effect, but a practical belief which is realized ? The very fact that it is practical means that it is translated into action ; it is almost tautology to say so ; and, furthermore, it tells us nothing concerning the mysterious character of this influence.

It thus would seem that M. F. Thomas was more exact in defining this general form of persuasion without apparent reason as " the inspiration of a belief the true

[1] *Education et hérédité*, Paris, p. 17.

motives of which escape us, and which tends of itself to be realized with more or less force ".[1]

Let us add two observations : First of all, if the foundations of this belief appear unknown at the actual moment of the suggestion, they need not have been so at a previous period of existence ; consciousness has thus preceded the unconscious. We thus again find that intermittence of consciousness, which is the distinctive sign of subconsciousness. The inspiration in question is an uprush of consciousness in a subconscious series. In the second place, this belief tends spontaneously to realization.

This essentially active character brings us back to the motor effects of ideas and images, that is to say, ideas by images. " Every idea is a force, and hence the commencement of an action. It always implies, in various degrees, an activity which tends to be exhibited, a power which tends towards an act, . . ." [2] " The thought," says Ribot, " is a word or act in the nascent state, that is to say, the beginning of muscular activity."

We see this dynamism of .the idea in the ordinary conditions of life, when the idea is fully conscious. Consider a child. Its physiognomy expresses its intimate states ; in its lively or clouded looks we discover the thought of joy or the feeling of sadness. At the end of a class, the idea of play about to begin is expressed by a certain agitation which is well known to teachers. There is no discontinuity between the idea and the movement which will be its normal expression : the idea is already the movement in its initial state. In the case of the adult, the watch which he keeps upon his attitudes allows the expression of the idea to be concealed up to a certain point. The idea nevertheless retains its motive power. " The greatest philosopher in the world," says Pascal, " standing on a plank of sufficient width, would find his

---

[1] Thomas (F.), *La suggestion, son rôle dans l'éducation*, Paris, pp. 20, 21.

[2] Fouillée, *Evolutionisme des idées-forces*, op. cit., *passim*.

imagination prevailing over him if suspended over a precipice, although his reason would convince him of his safety. There are many who could not entertain the thought without turning pale and perspiring." [1] The sight of the precipice suggests the idea of a possible fall, and this idea by its own dynamism, tends to make us fall.

Chevreul carried out an experiment with a pendulum which confirms this theory. Taking the pendulum in his hand he thought of its possible movements, and the thought alone was sufficient to produce oscillatory movements. He followed with his eyes these oscillations and saw their amplitude increase. Thus perception alone increased the vivacity of the idea and hence its motive power.

After preservation in the memory and recall, the idea has not lost its power of movement. "We cannot," says Joly, "remember a musical air without a kind of weak vibration seeming, like a distant echo, to cause our ear to vibrate, to the point of imperceptible movements of the head and body, which beat the time."

Other facts seem to confirm this motive influence of the memory at the moment of its recall. We recollect a disagreeable taste, and immediately we are strongly affected by it and feel sick. We have a delicious dish placed in front of us, and experience its delightful taste in anticipation. As Taine says, the image of the expected taste is equivalent to the sensation of present taste ; the resemblance goes so far that, in both cases, the salivary glands secrete to the same extent. We have already studied the subconscious mechanisms, and it may be asked for what reason we now return to them.

It is for the reason that unconscious dynamism, properly so called, begins at the frontier of automatism. We must guard against believing reality to be discontinuous and distinct when it actually forms an uninterrupted series. We thus unite these two types of phenomena with one

---

[1] Quoted by F. Thomas, op cit., p. 6.

another, since the second is the design amplified by sketches made by the first.

In the case of auto-suggestion, dynamism is clearly distinguished from the automatic mechanism which precedes it, and of which it is a prolongation.

In the course of a reverie, my glance falls upon the design of a fabric or the arabesques of an oriental temple. Up to a point, I experience very ordinary sensations and perceptions, but suddenly I find that an original image appears before my eyes. The design is transformed into a face, the arabesques represent a person. The illusion is so perfect that the same transformation will be repeated later when the perception is renewed. Thus an image has aroused one greater than itself, an idea has excited the production of another more complex.

What has happened ? At a given moment in my life, I saw Turkish figures at the entrance to a mosque. They were certainly different from the arabesques which the Islamic artists had drawn on the walls of their house of prayer. But under favourable circumstances these two images, the Turk's head and the geometrical design, which at first were close to one another, became one. Something took place in my imagination analogous to the digestion of images. Thus, as the result of this unconscious work, my two ideas, originally distinct, were adapted and assimilated to the point of absorbing one another. We thus have here an original creation, produced by auto-suggestion, together with the mechanism by which the idea was exteriorized.

In the preceding example, it was the observation of nature which was the immediate cause of an entirely unexpected mental development. Very many scientists have found in this way the theme of their brilliant theories. Malus, Niepce, Ampère, Pasteur made investigations ; their observations were followed by reflective work. Then, after a certain period of rest, they returned to their idea and found it enlarged and, as it were, metamorphosed.

Often also, meditation upon reading produced this amplification. Descartes read the scholastics ; Leibniz read Fermat and Pascal, perhaps even Newton, but certainly Descartes ; Pascal was informed of the researches of Galilei and learnt the result of Torricelli's experiment. All these seekers made use of their documents in elaborating their new theories. As the guardian of the ideas of others and the revelation of the valuable scientific acquisitions of the past, the book is like a prolonged observation ; it even tends to assume, in the permanence of its well-ordered pages, a kind of eternal character. It can be meditated upon at leisure and used as a guide.

The combined results of observation and reading produce the effect which Schopenhauer calls " unconscious rumination ". " It is the rumination of thoughts," says J. Jastrow, " that prepares them for assimilation by our mental tissues." [1] This work is, in fact, an assimilation. Now, in the physiological domain this transformation is unconscious, but no one would, however, deny its existence. From the certainty of the effect the certainty of the invisible cause may be concluded. We may thus be allowed to reason in the same way in psychology. If the fact of these mental modifications is certain, the invisible cause is not less so.

This progress of victorious thought implies the meeting of ideas, the reduction of some, the amplification of others ; in short, it implies a latent dynamism in the association of ideas.

III. The Dynamic Unconscious Effects the Association of Ideas

The association of ideas is generally pictured as taking place in an inert reservoir in which our ideas are passively preserved, but grouped into distinct bundles. There are three serious errors in this view. (1) The function in question is the power which ideas have of

---

[1] Jastrow, *La subsconscience*, p. 69.

suggesting one another; consequently it should be called the evocation or the suggestion of images. (2) It is an essentially *active* faculty, it is the tendency which our mind has to pass spontaneously from one idea to another. (3) It is not a fate reserved for ideas alone ; all states of consciousness, ideas, images, sensations, internal movements are ruled by the same law. On the other hand, since this power is exercized between phenomena different in nature, between feelings and ideas, feelings and volitions, all psychological phenomena which are conscious, are influenced by this drive of suggestion and reciprocal evocation. Finally, unconscious psychical facts also feel the effect of it, since, as we have seen in the Introduction, a fully conscious emotion would seem isolated and remain inexplicable if it had not been suggested by an unconscious factor. We thus find in the association of psychical states a powerful dynamism which explains all the various orientations of thought and feeling.

Psychologists tell us that it acts by the laws of *contiguity*, of *resemblance*, of *transference* and of *contrast*. It is easy to prove that the law of contrast may be reduced to that of resemblance, for contraries represent the extreme terms of the same genus ; hence, by virtue of some relation, they are similar ; black and white are both colours, sweet and bitter are both tastes.

In the same way, the law of transference is only a derived form of that of resemblance. In fact, if two representations have been associated and if a feeling accompanies one of them, it is also attached to the other. This feeling is thus the element of likeness which links the two representations together.

Finally, contiguity sums up all the other laws, it has been said, because in order to be associated, like elements must be brought together in the same consciousness.

Does the reduction cease at this point ? Why does the contiguity of two ideas suffice for one to be evoked by the other ? This previous contiguity in consciousness, whether total or partial, mediate or immediate, simultaneous or successive, would not produce association if there were not a kind of partial identity, of possible bond, between the elements to be united. Let us make this point clear. It is not a question of fusing together all the elements of which an associated group is composed. It is simply necessary to explain by a sufficient reason the fact of their mutual evocation, at a given moment, in the same consciousness.

What is this attraction but the attraction exercised between psychical elements ?   But this attraction has no other reason for existence than community of origin. The sun attracts the planets because the planets are derived from the sun ; the earth attracts the moon because this satellite is like a bud derived from the world which we inhabit ; the mother attracts her child by the bond of her natural affection because, as Aristotle says, the child is something of its mother.

Thus if an idea or an image arouses a procession of other ideas or other images in consciousness, it is because, according to the law formulated by Hoffding, " Every fact of consciousness which is reproduced tends to restore the total state of which it forms a part." Thus every evocative idea forms part of a group ; it is by virtue of being the part of a whole, one element, of a collection, that it has this attractive power. Its dynamism, whether it be known or unknown, conscious or unconscious, is thus the result of its relations with the group. It is in this sense that we understand this partial identity. It is indeed a form of assimilation, since the idea called upon to integrate itself in a group is only classed in this group as part of a collection, as an element of a whole. Nevertheless, association is not synthesis. These ideas called together to a meeting, are only stones awaiting the construction of the building. They all have characters in common, and this similarity makes possible an alliance which is not yet consummated, but is prepared for.

Judgment and reason will cement it. For the moment,

it is sufficient to note the attraction which has brought
the ideas together. It may be objected that this energy
is purely imaginary, and that the will has caused them
to be brought together. But this cannot be the case, since
the will depends upon the intelligence, whereas the first
origin of the association was unconscious. The force in
question is thus distinct from the will.

The rôle of this latent dynamism is not, however,
limited to promoting the reunion of ideas nor to
constituting groups or images. The mind is essentially
active, and transforms its psychical groupings at every
moment, decomposes and recomposes them, dissociates
and associates them. The attractive force that we have
regarded as the origin of association has not expended
its creative power. We find it in the service of the
imagination as well, the supreme combining faculty.

IV. The Dynamic Unconscious Effects the Constructive Work of the Creative Imagination

Every inventive genius is more or less a seer, a kind
of prophet of science. He sees in the present, he utilizes
the gifts of the past, and he reads the future, thanks to that
marvellous producer of images, the imagination. With
the help of it, Newton passed from the observation of a
falling apple to the vision of universal attraction. Watt
saw Newcomen's engine, and caught a glimpse of his
own condenser. In the case of all these constructors of
genius, progress is accomplished, a step forward is made ;
there is a powerful urge in them to do better than their
predecessors. They all seem to have their eyes fixed
upon an ideal image, and the programme which they
set out to accomplish has been laid down for them by
the imagination.

In fact, as Ribot writes, " the representation of a movement is a movement beginning." Now it is the imagination that produces the representation : " The imagination

is thus, in the intellectual order, the equivalent of the will in the order of movements."

Its dynamism excites the apparition of the novel image under the form of a sudden illumination which has been prepared in the unconscious ; for, as Ribot, quoting Dubois-Reymond, says : " I have had in my life a few happy discoveries, and I have often remarked that they came when I was not thinking about it." "That little electric shock which strikes you in the head " is inspiration.[1]

What is the nature of this force ? It is painful in some cases, agreeable in others. It is an urge which is superior to the individual consciousness, for the latter author says in his confidences : " *I* don't count in it at all."

It implies, first of all, the concentration of the faculties upon a single point. In itself, " it is a cerebration or activity of a purely physiological nature, or a gradual diminution of the consciousness which exists without being united with the ego, that is, the principal consciousness."

But this inspiration differs from paramnesia. In false memory, there is a rapid succession of two perceptions, one of which, hardly noticed, takes on the character of a recollection, but there are no new combinations. This stamp of novelty is always found in inspirations.

On the other hand, this vigour of thought cannot be confused with that which precedes intoxication. In the latter, indeed, the directive principle which imposes unity, is wanting. Inspiration, on the contrary, while remaining a progress in ideas, is attached to the thread of past reasoning by a powerful bond.

Since it is the idea in action, Ribot believes that it is to be assimilated to certain forms of somnambulism ; it would be "somnambulism in a waking state, but in less degree ". At normal times, conscious activity outshines by its clarity our unconscious activity. By a reversal of order," Inspiration would be unconscious activity passing

[1] Ribot, *L'imagination créatrice*, p. 44.

T

to the first plane ; it would be like a cipher telegram transmitted by unconscious activity to conscious activity." [1]

This ingenious comparison well expresses the unexpected character of inspiration. But there is nothing pathological in this inversion of somnambulism ; it represents a normal phase of intellectual life ; it makes known the precise moment at which an idea, grafted upon a group of other ideas, is revealed to consciousness with its original shade of meaning. This process is as regular as the discontinuous discharge of water from intermittent geysers. The invisible ascent of the water from the earth is admitted to be regular. There is no reason for regarding the appearance of the liquid at the surface, once the required level has been obtained, as an abnormal phenomenon. Now inspiration is nothing else than a spurt of psychical life passing from the unconscious to the conscious plane. Consequently the latent dynamism which prepares the invention, acts through a regular process.

On the other hand, is this sublimal activity merely unconscious cerebration ? It is impossible to admit this. For inventive work implies the adaptation of ideas to other ideas, corrections, rational operations. How then could nervous modifications alone cause an original idea to be produced ? If they are modified by memory they do not themselves modify memories. We must thus have recourse to a psychical factor in order to explain the point of departure of the invention.

Now, if we consult our everyday experience, we see that there is a parallelism between our conscious and our unconscious activity. When playing the piano, whether I think of the notes or whether, the tune being known to me, I allow my fingers to move over the keys without reflection, the result is identical. When writing a letter I sometimes pay attention to the words I am

---

[1] Ribot, op. cit., p. 47 ; Chabaneix, *Le subconscient chez les artistes, les savants, et les ecrivains*, p. 87.

using and sometimes I am simply preoccupied with the thought to be expressed, and allow the pen to trace by habit the signs which correspond to my ideas. In both cases, I find on re-reading the letter that both writing and orthography are equally good. Up to this point, we are in the domain of automatism. We may simply conclude that acts done by habit do not differ essentially from those done with reflection.

We may go further and assume the intervention of the dynamic unconscious. I seek the solution of a problem and after various combinations effected in full consciousness, I find it. The next day I propose to solve a similar but more difficult problem. Various trials are unsuccessful. I cease for the moment to pursue my labour, I go for a walk, and suddenly, at a moment when I was not thinking of the matter, the happy combination appears in my mind, evoked by some association of ideas or other. On verification it is found to be the solution.

In both cases, there is a certain equivalence. The facts demonstrate that the dynamism of ideas is up to a certain point, which we shall define more precisely later, independent of consciousness. It is a psychical constant.

Can the reason prove this sufficiently ? The problem comes back to this : does the unitive, synthetic, assimilative power of ideas come from consciousness, and does it come from consciousness alone ?

Let us first of all note that ideas do not function without images. Now these are the work of the imagination. But this creative power of the universe, when regarded in the potential or pure state, entirely escapes consciousness. There is thus a radical unconscious at the origin of all images.

Furthermore, the image is attached to a sensation and a movement ; this connection, indeed, is what gives it its true physiognomy. Now we are never conscious of this point of attachment, and when we discover it by analysis, it is already formed. We come on the scene after the fact is accomplished.

Finally, if the image is essentially the generator of movement, its activity is not conditioned by consciousness. More than this : the gaze of the mind is able to hinder its flight, if not to paralyse it. To be conscious, in fact, is to reflect, to compare, to weigh pros and cons, and thus is in the first place to retard action, and often also, as a result of this preliminary deliberation, to weaken its vigour.

Following Ribot, we have established a relationship between inspiration and somnambulism. But in the case of the sleep-walking neurotic, whence is his surety in the execution of an act derived if not from the unabated power of the idea directing him, of the image which seems to afford him the light of an inward vision ?

Thus, considered by itself, the image is possessed of its own virtue : it can do without consciousness.

However, this is only part of the truth. While the image, in transforming itself into movement, does no more than exhibit externally the powers concealed in it, it is certain that, at a given moment, it is reinforced and amplified by a certain tonality received from consciousness. One might even say that it has been prepared in the warm sun of consciousness. It was certainly with a knowledge of their motive that Ampère, Fresnel, Watt, Poincaré furnished their minds with the elements which they were to integrate in the inventions of their genius.

The essential work of the imagination is to dissociate in order to make new associations. But we perform these two operations without thinking about it ; it is after the event, by reflection, that we become aware of the results of this decomposition followed by recomposition. For example, when Newton dissociated the idea of the movement of a falling apple to associate it with that of the moon revolving around our planet, he effected this analysis and synthesis without thinking of anything else but the result he was pursuing. In the same way, Lavoisier brought together by his imagination rust, combustion, and respiration.   How can we imagine that phenomena so far apart could be grouped together intentionally by a man of genius ?   The ideas gathered concerning this question were united among themselves unconsciously, by virtue of their own power.

In order to reinforce this immanent power of the imagination, founded on the reciprocal influence of body and mind, brain workers have put themselves in the best organic condition to create in the endeavour to produce a high degree of vital tone, they have made use of artificial procedures, the strangeness of which would cause us to smile, were we not aware of their hidden motive.   In order to increase the flow of blood to the brain, Rousseau worked with his head uncovered in full sunshine.   Boussuet, on the contrary, remained in a cold room with his head wrapped up.   Schiller kept his feet in cold water ; Descartes and Leibniz placed themselves in an almost horizontal position ; Lamennais walked about and followed his thoughts in the midst of the noise of festivals as well as in silence and darkness.[1] On the other hand, we already know that H. Poincaré, when seeking the solution of the problem of fuchsian functions, discovered it after having taken a double portion of strong black coffee on the evening before ; in this respect he followed the example of the Goncourts, who sought the hyperæsthesia favourable to literary inspiration in the abuse of wine and tobacco, of coffee, and late hours.   As Ribot says, they were convinced of the profound analogy between invention and physical creation, which is a " prolonged nutrition ", and sought a superabundance of psychical life in order to ensure their imaginative constructions.

This imaginative energy, according as it is intuitive or combinative, modifies the inventive mind and confers upon it, according to Ribot, a well-characterized scientific direction.   When it is intuitive, and grafted on an

[1] Ribot, *L'imagination créatrice*, p. 65.

inductive mind, it produces the observer, the naturalist, the psychologist. When it is intuitive and associated with a deductive intelligence, it gives us the naturalist and geometor. When it is combinative, in association with an inductive mind, we have the industrialist, the technician, and, in another region, the poet and the artist. When it appears in a combinative form in a deductive mind, we have the mathematician, if deduction is predominant, and the philosopher, if imagination is preponderant. In every case, a latent dynamism is at the base of all progress. Is this mysterious power manifested only in the creation of images ? We believe that it expands a still greater amount of energy in the synthesis of our judgments.

V. The Synthetic Unconscious

In reality, it is in this form that the idea, preserved in the potential state, manifests its full creative vigour. In order to convince ourselves of this, let us examine its power as revealed in the light of consciousness, and then proceed to inquire whether its virtue ceases to be operative when it passes into the unconscious state. Let us take an example.

I have studied and compared with one another all systems of morality. Little by little, confronting all these theories with the characters of necessity and universality required for moral obligation, I have clearly seen that the pursuit of the rational good can alone form the foundation of morality. During this progress of my thought, I have noted those phases which were completely conscious ; in such cases, the progress of my ideas was clearly perceived, and consequently brought into quick correlation with the value of these ideas. Their power was thus a fully illuminated power.

But I also noted the existence of moments of relative unconsciousness. How was it that, after having ceased to compare various systems of ethics, I found one day that I possessed firm convictions upon this question. I perceived that I had made great progress during this slumber of reflection. For the idea, preserved in memory, had kept its effective power, had preserved its coefficient of development. Whether I perceive it or not, the psychical state which I carry within me is thus, like a volcano, continually active. Whether conscious or not, my intellectual modifications proceed to evolve in my inward laboratory. My thought remains always active ; it improves, it annexes new elements when I leave it to itself ; it then returns to me laden with unsuspected property. What I thus observe in myself is the same fact that the great constructors of systems noticed in themselves. Newton, Leibniz, Pascal, Cuvier, Darwin, Pasteur and many others ripened their ideas little by little, without perceiving the fact at the most decisive moment. This logical unconscious, which presides over the formation of our deepest convictions, which co-ordinates our mental acquisitions into an harmonious synthesis, which ensures at every moment the progress of our thought, is a hidden force. It is impossible not to recognize its existence if we insist on accounting for this incessant ripening of our ideas. But how are we to explain it ? Is it not quite simply an application of the psychological law : resemblances reinforce one another, differences annul one another ? When working in the full light of consciousness, we effect numerous reductions in the mass of representations which encumber our minds ; we strive to retain only what is essential. Consequently, our memory concentrates its activity upon this limited field of recollections. The result is that these latter acquire an excess vivacity ; they are less numerous but more active.

Why should not this dynamism continue its activity when we are not thinking about it ? Facts prove that this is the case. But then the same cause should produce the same effect. If psychical states retain during sleep an activity of which we are ignorant, it is because they have retained the dynamism of the waking state. In the same way, if the synthetic connection, which in the sequel will be expressed in the form of judgment, is effected without the help of consciousness, it must be that the spiritual force producing linkage during the phase of unconscious activity is of the same nature as that which brings it about in the full light of reflection.

We may go further. This synthetic organization of our judgments is often produced with greater surety when we are not thinking about it than when our mind follows the logical development with a critical eye. The very numerous facts which we have brought together as proof in the first part of this study, establish it to the full. What is the reason for this superiority of unconscious labour ? It is this : that in the reflective preparation of a conclusion, ideas of opposing force successively pass in review and are valued according to ordinary procedure ; the idea most highly rated in this comparative examination is not the most original one. We reason in accordance with our past reasoning. The result is first of all a waste of time, and then a conclusion which does not dare to be an invention ; in the course of strictly conscious reasoning, the mind with its well-formed habits reasons in accordance with these habits. This results in a kind of intellectual routine and a rarity of discoveries in the case of minds which are exclusively deductive and too systematic. On the contrary, during unconscious activity, the excess value of an idea—preserved in the form of a mental state—takes effect without suffering the competition of rival idea of less importance, because these latter are eliminated by themselves. Hence the fertile idea, the idea rich in promise, the idea which will form the scientist's hypothesis, arrives straight away, without the delay imposed by criticism, at its linkage with another, a linkage which, in the form of an intuition, will be suddenly revealed to consciousness. That is why, in accordance with the penetrating remark of Souriau. " It is necessary to think off the mark " in order to discover and invent. To think off the mark is, at a given moment to abandon the logical track previously traced out, in order to attempt to link up an idea which has come to us suddenly, an idea which is strange at first sight, an idea thrown from the subconscious into the consciousness by reason of an observation or experiment.   The mind then proceeds like a young man who, in the hope of a fortunate marriage, leaves his environment, his caste, sometimes even his native country, to form an alliance with a young foreigner. This kind of marriage is, we are assured, the most fertile. Hence these combinations of psychical elements derived, some from a conscious source, others from a subconscious centre, give promise of the most numerous, if not always the most beautiful inventions.

VI. SUMMARY AND CONCLUSION

Finally, therefore, the dynamic unconscious appears to us in the form of a suggestion or belief which strives to realize itself without a plausible motive.   We have thus returned to the motive effect of ideas by way of images, an effect which we have already analysed in the study of the automatic unconscious.   Then, passing beyond this point of view, we have seen the psychical transformation and enlargement effected by the latent power of ideas.   This extension implied an association, and hence a certain assimilation of ideas.   But these ideas do not operate without images.   We thus pass from association to that great purveyor of ideas, the imagination.   But an image and a combination of images do not suffice ; an unconscious synthetic activity allows of the progressive formation of our most original judgments by the adoption of ideas which our logical mind would, perhaps, have disowned, if these new arrivals had been presented to it through the channel of conscious reflection.

In the suggestion of the idea, in its association with other ideas, in its imaginative transformations, and in the synthetic linkage of judgments, a dynamism, hidden but real, thus governs the activity of the mind.

All the same, while demonstrating this fact with the fullest evidence, we have not yet explained the mystery of discoveries and inventions. At ordinary times, during the conscious phases of our thought, " the motive force of the idea varies in accordance with the affective element to which it is united." [1] The idea is only fertile when it is supported by the feeling. On the other hand, we have remarked with Abramowski that the majority of mental images, disappearing from the field of consciousness, are preserved in the lower psychism in the form of feeling. It thus seems logical to inquire whether it is not precisely in this affective form that our past representations have preserved their dynamic value. While active in the fully conscious state, they owed their energetic tonality to their emotional coefficient. When active in the state of unconscious residues, they should in the same way remain operative by virtue of feeling. Our study of unconscious dynamism in the genesis of invention thus leads us to a necessary complement : the analysis of the rôle played by the æsthetic unconscious.

[1] Thomas, op. cit., p. 8.

CHAPTER IV

THE ROLE OF THE ÆSTHETIC UNCONSCIOUS IN INVENTION

The constant necessity for the association of feeling with the fertile idea—The survival of feeling in the idea is possible—The characters of the effective unconscious—The fertility of the æsthetic unconscious—The transition from the unconscious to consciousness—Summary and conclusion.

IN order to continue its mental transformations, the idea, in ceasing to be conscious, cannot perish entirely ; it must continue to act in the form of feeling.

We thus have to investigate the necessity, the possibility, the characteristics, and the fertility of this survival of the idea in a more or less unconscious form. Passing, finally, from twilight to the full light of consciousness, we shall see the precious products of these affective metamorphoses in inventive incubation.

I. THE CONSTANT NECESSITY FOR THE ASSOCIATION OF FEELING WITH THE IDEA

We have seen that the motive power of the idea varies in the same way as the affective element with which it is associated.

Every day experience proves this. Ideas which interest us are those capable of holding our attention. Other ideas, which are accompanied by no emotion, leave no traces on our minds. This is, however, only part of the truth. We may note first of all, with Thomas, " that it is not purely animal sensations which act most powerfully upon us, but rather feelings which envelop an intellectual representation, image or idea, which is more clear and precise." [1]

[1] Thomas (F.), *La suggestion, son rôle dans l'éducation*, p. 11

On the other hand, in many cases feeling does not excite activity. When it is excessive, it paralyses action ; when it is suddenly produced, it suspends it ; when it occurs unawares it causes confusion in the mind instead of illuminating it.

Finally, certain feelings, far from being energetic factors are essentially depressing ; mistrust, apprehension, terror, obscure the mind and, instead of exciting moral struggle, accelerate defeat. On the other hand, we find in confidence and hope a new lease of life, and an increase in power.

Before considering the efficaciousness of feeling in producing an invention, we need, first of all, to take into consideration both the relative intensity, the sudden or progressive appearance, and the nature of these psychical states.

Between these emotive tendencies a battle is fought ; the conquered disappear at least momentarily from the field of battle, the victors make use to their profit of the movement which has brought them into being. It is from this internal conflict that the habitual happiness or fundamental sadness which characterizes us, according to the issue of the battle, proceeds. Victory is always due to the predominance of one feeling over others.

Thus, given a conscious psychical state, the feeling and the idea are associated. The feeling supports the idea, fertilizes it, and translates it into action.

This characteristic dualism of a psychical state is found again in considering this state as past and in its relations with a present state.

Rignano has put this in a clear light : " The conscious character of a past psychical state, in relation to a present psychical state, is always met with whenever we have coexistence for a certain time of the former with the latter, and the superposition or fusion of one with the other. It is, however, necessary that this superposition and partial fusion should be produced in the affective part played of the two psychical states."

The same author shows us the way in which the fusion is effected, as follows :—

" These cerebral zones, to the activity of which these psychical states, the one evoked, the other actual, are due, come into coincidence, or into juxtaposition in respect of a certain common portion only . . . In parallel with the series of our conscious actions, corresponding complex affective states always succeed one another, such that each, commencing its activity before the cessation of the preceding act, is subsequently continuous during the two first stages or the complete development of the following act, and sometimes during a whole series of successive acts. Such an affective state is a bond of union. A meeting is desired : this desire for a meeting continues during the whole series of acts which have for their aim to bring it about. The same is true of every example which we could give. In these various cases, what is unconscious is sometimes " internal meditation " and sometimes " the series of sensations aroused by the external world ".[1]

This relation is true of conscious states, and not less so of unconscious. The following is the way in which Rignano perceives this relationship between conscious and unconscious psychical states.

" Every psychical state by itself is neither conscious nor unconscious. But it becomes one or the other through its relationship to some other psychical state . . . Consciousness is the character of a relationship between several psychical states. Consciousness is an extrinsic and relative property of psychical states.[2]

II. THE SURVIVAL OF FEELING IN THE IDEA IS POSSIBLE

Among the facts which prove this are several referred to by Dr. Herbert in his work on *Auto-Suggestion.*

[1] Rignano (E.), *Essai de synthèse scientifique*, Paris, 1912, p. 158.
[2] Op. cit., p. 164.

" The mental impression," he writes, " may be made voluntarily, for example, if I impress upon my mind the thought that I must get up at a certain time in the morning ; or the impression may be made involuntarily ; in this case it is the result of a series of ideas awakened unconsciously by some external influence or by a corporeal sensation of real or imaginary origin. For example, a man may have touched a garment and, learning that it had been worn by a person suffering from skin disease, he immediately begins to feel itching all over his body and imagines that he has contracted the disease . . ."

" Many phenomena attributed to intuition may be caused by involuntary auto-suggestion. Thus a child may take a dislike to a man who has spoken harshly or committed a base act in its presence. The man and the incident may have been completely forgotten, but the impression is stored in that marvellous recording apparatus, the mind, and, years afterwards, the child, now a man, will experience aversion for everybody resembling the man whom he detested in his childhood, and this dislike will persist. .If your ask anyone who experiences such an antipathy why he detests a person to whom he has just been introduced, he will probably say to you : ' Oh, I don't know why I don't like him, but I know that I detest him. My antipathy for him is instinctive.' And all the same this antipathy is not instinctive. It is the result of an involuntary suggestion arising from impressions stored up in infancy and awakened by a series of fortuitous thoughts aroused by a single glance at a new face."

In these various cases, the idea is forgotten, the intellectual phenomenon has passed to the state of an unconscious residue, but the emotional phenomenon has been preserved in a certain way. The fact of this affective continuity may thus be considered as assured.

Let us see what is the mode of operation of this extinction of consciousness in favour of an affective state, which has become a kind of universal legatee.

Abramowski has made numerous experiments on the two parts of memory : the image part, in strict relationship with the activity of the intellect ; and the undifferentiated and non-representative or non-intellectual part which we feel as " the consciousness of a gap " in reproduction and as the feeling of the already known in recognition.

Following this author, we can distinguish four degrees in this non-intellectual consciousness of recollection: (1) " The lowest ˉdegree is the consciousness of a gap in description . . . It is an indetermined feeling that something is wanting, and an immediate knowledge not inferred, and without any intelligible reason, that there is a forgotten part about which we can say nothing."

(2) If we bring this consciousness of something wanting into the act of comparison with things different from the forgotten matter we are seeking, we then see that it is not only a general consciousness of something wanting, but that it offers a certain more or less strong resistance to false suggestions, and does not allow the gaps which are felt to be filled indifferently by anything : this is the second degree of non-intellectual consciousness of recollection: the generic or specific feeling of the gap. Here, just as in the preceding case, the knowledge that " it is not this " is immediate and not reasoned ; we do not know why the forgotten detail is not this or that, but we have an intuitive certainty in feeling.

(3) On theˉother hand, if instead of comparing the forgotten thing with different things, we present to the subject the forgotten thing itself, the perception of this thing is then (if forgetfulness is not complete) accompanied by a specific feeling of recognition, of repetition, a feeling which is entirely ˉpositive to our introspection ; this is the third degree of non-intellectual consciousness of recollection. Here also the knowledge " that has already been " is immediate and not reasoned. We ordinarily recognize at first sight without evoking the past.

(4) " The last degree of the non-intellectual consciousness of recollection, the strongest and that presenting
an infinite emotional variation, is manifested in the
symbolism of words and images, in so far as they are
recollections. In the terms themselves which designate
persons, places, things or events, even when they are
not accompanied by any image, there is a certain manner
of feeling the words, an emotional stamp on each word,
which gives it the value of a concrete recollection and
distinguishes it from those which are not the symbol
of past experience. In our thoughts and associations,
we react quite specially to these recollection words,
although in the actual perception of the symbolic term,
apart from the visual and audio-motive elements of the
sign, there is nothing but this emotional colour,
imperceptible to thought, but which the past speaks to
us. When such a sign is received, we are already in
possession of the recollection, even before images and
associations rise up . . ."

" The definition of a recollection best fitting results
of experience would be as follows : the total recollection
is an affective phenomenon partially intellectualized
in images." [1]

In another passage, the same psychologist defines the
place of the affective phenomenon in relation to the
impression and the image, and thus formulates his theory
of recognition :—

" In the act of recognition, the recollection is joined
to the impression before it develops into an image, that
is to say, it is joined in its a-intellectual aspect, which is
rather affective than representative. In fusing with the
impression, it gives this an emotional colour. It
impregnates it with a specific feeling of identity or
novelty, which, at the first moment of perception, does
not yet constitute an object of distinct thought of the
impression, but forms with the latter one and the same
perception.

---

[1] Abramowski, *Le subconscient normal*, pp. 22, 23–4.

This emotional stamp of the impression is the point of departure and the basis of the judgment of recognition. It is only in the following phase that it is separated from the impression, develops into an image, and constitutes the intellectual act of comparison made up of two terms, the memory image and external perception. Recognition is thus the perception of an object under its a-intellectual aspect ; it is an affective phenomenon, a feeling of familiarity incorporated with the impression.[1]

Abramowski defines his thought more exactly, and deduces from his experiments the progressive substitution of the affective state for perception considered in its intellectual phase :—

" In every perception there are two elements : the pure impression, that is to say, the immediate expression of the active environment, and its intellectual elaboration resulting from the act of attention, as in states of mental distraction ; it then constitutes a psychical state which is a-intellectual and undetermined for thought, an uncertain and anonymous mode of feeling which may almost be expressed introspectively by the general judgment : " that something has been there." It is a perception reduced to the state of a certain kind of feeling. The act of attention transforms this something of indeterminate or emotional nature into an object of definite thought, capable of being named, into a perception capable of being identified and classed, and of forming judgments, the equivalents of which are found in language. Perception reduced to an indeterminate state of feeling is, for our intellect, the " subconscious ", inaccessible to thought, although psychical and influencing thought.

(2) " When perception passes into forgetfulness it produces for the latter a like emotional reduction. The forgotten is preserved, not only physiologically as a residual modification of the brain, but also psychically as a subconscious state, as the emotional equivalent of a past perception. Under this aspect, it is manifested to us

---

[1] Op. cit., p. 49.

introspectively and experimentally in the act of inhibited
recollection. (The feeling of the forgotten is expressed
by the current phrase " It's on the tip of my tongue ".)
In the resistance which the thing forgotten opposes to
incorrect recollection ('although I cannot remember
what it is, I know it is not that ') ; in the feeling of
recognition which is the evocation by perception of its
previous emotional reduction ; in the hallucinations of
memory in which this reduction, preserved in forgetfulness,
finds an erroneous but emotionally similar expression ;
finally, in paramnesias, in which the emotional reduction
produced at the very moment of perception, by a double
vision of the thing, plays the part of the forgotten and
produces in the case of something new the illusion of its
being something from the past."

(3) " It would follow from this that in the psychical
world nothing perishes and that all the past of the
individual, the whole mass of forgotten things, which
is reproduced in conscious recollection only partially
and from time to time, exists constantly and as a whole
in the form of an enormous, uniform, subconscious memory
store, not differentiated by thought, in the state of the
emotional reduction of the past . . . Every moment lived
through leaves behind its emotional equivalent, a vestige
preserved in the unconscious, of its past existence ; and
thus our ' ego ' is gradually created : *the past actually
in existence.*

"Sometimes we differentiate these relics by the
activity of our thought, we resuscitate fragmentarily
as conscious and definite recollection ; but in a
subconscious fashion, anonymously, emotionally,
remember them always, inasmuch as they form an
undifferentiated element constituting the feeling of
our own ego." [1]

The affective state thus survives the representative
state : the feeling prolongs the idea ; the feeling and the
idea, associated in consciousness, are not absolutely

[1] Op. cit., pp. 136, 137.

separated in the unconscious : one inherits from the other, feeling succeeds provisionally to the idea, we thus have an emotional unconscious. What are its characters ?

III. THE CHARACTERS OF THE AFFECTIVE UNCONSCIOUS

First of all, as we have just seen, this emotional state produced from unconscious tendencies, pure memory devoid of all representative element, is the mysterious reverberation of all that we have lived through. Consequently, considering only its origin, we should discover in its content a complexity of elements to explain partially the diversity of its characters. Being in relationship with the organism by cenesthesia, it constitutes a kind of defence of it ; organic influences act upon conscious feelings through its intervention.

Being inseparable from the activity of the subject the æsthetic unconscious is associated ; it connects among themselves individual attitudes and transformation. It links together groups of ideas, modifies them, makes tendencies of them, and gives them durability and stability.

Now tendencies organize themselves, and seek the justification of ideas : hence the affective state which has produced them and which supports them influences the formation of judgments.[1] Regarded under this aspect, the unconscious is the " affective status memory " of Ribot ; it is also the " affective dynamic memory " or the reproductive memory. Ribot doubts the existence of the latter ; he is wrong. It is necessary in order to prolong the preservative action of the first.

At the same time as being a substitute for feeling or passion, the affective unconscious also assumes the impulsive form. In this case, it has a less intensity, but greater persistence, than the conscious feeling.

[1] Cf. Dwelshauvers, *L'inconscient*, pp. 112, 194 et seq.

All the same, the coefficient of activity depends upon the preceding idea, of which the unconscious feeling is regarded as being the psychical heir. Consequently we may agree with A. Fouillée in distinguishing four degrees, as it were, four cases in this dynamism of the unconscious affective state.

(1) A simple idea caused by the excitation of nervous centres always produces an emotional reaction.

(2) When it is intense, lively, clear, it produces a more intense and lively emotion.

(3) The force of the emotion is greater if the idea includes a more distinct representation of movement, and if it is more easily reducible to movement.

(4) The idea and the emotion are easily suggested if the movements are depicted by the imagination.

Such are the relations between ideas and feeling during the conscious phase. There follows the period of unconsciousness in which the affective state perceives representations; this state will remain proportional to the intellectual cause which gave birth to it; it will thus be more active the clearer the generative idea was, the greater the content of movement in the generative representation, and the more richly the motive idea is surrounded by imagery, produced by the efforts of the imagination.

On the other hand, adds Fouillée, "in the loss of memories, feelings disappear after ideas, but before automatic acts . . . Memory properly so-called is in feeling; it is there that the most resistance is offered, after automatic acts." Thus if we accept this point, the ideas of this philosopher, it is under the form of the *automatic* unconscious and of the *affective* unconscious that psychical force—that is to say the capacity for original creation—has the greatest chance of being conserved.

Now we have seen that, in spite of its utility, automatism alone is incapable of invention. Consequently, when representative phenomena have disappeared into the unconscious, it is clearly in the affective form that they are most susceptible to creative and lasting transformation.[1]

It is this continued efficacy of the emotional residue which we are now going to examine.

IV. The Fertility of the Æsthetic Unconscious

Abramowski has thus summed up his experiments on paramnesia and recognition :—

" The degree of mobility or, in other words, of spontaneous creation, of the subconscious depends upon the extent of its affective kindred, and upon the associated ramifications which depend to a great extent upon it. If this affective kindred is poor, or if the associated routes are functionally inhibited (which may happen from different causes) the conditions are then not favourable to unconscious transformations. The points of contact between the subconscious and the intellectual synthetic consciousness are less numerous ; the possibility of modifying influences which may proceed from it is at its maximum ; we almost have a dissociation. Conversely the subconscious state which finds in the organism a rich affective kindred and free associative paths, remains within the sphere of the influences of the intellectual consciousness, and, without yet issuing from its cryptamnesia, is able to be transformed ; it is creative before becoming conscious." [2]

This assertion is not gratuitous : Abramowski proves by a series of experiments that this unconscious transformation operates precisely because the requisite conditions—affective kindred, points of contact with the intellectual consciousness, freedom of associated paths— are frequently realized. In this case, we not only have

---

[1] Fouillée, *Psychologie des idées-forces*, i, p. 205.
[2] Op. cit., p. 151.

conservation of the invisible mental state, but modification and creative progression. The following is a summary of the results of these experiments.

As memory object, he used "illustrated postcards showing compositions with different amounts of detail perceived under different conditions.

"The experiment consisted in two descriptions of each card. The first followed immediately upon perception. The subject sketched on the paper what he had seen, and at the same time related, in all its details, the design copied from memory. The design was made in an altogether formalized manner. This was repeated after each of six perceptions. There was thus obtained in this way the first mental image, the image in its primitive phase, still closely in contact with its origin."

"After a week, a second description of each card was made in the same manner, with the help of drawing and detailed narration. This was the second mental image, which gave, as compared with the first, the cryptamnesic history of each perception, the history of the subconscious state during a week of its latent life. The subject was not forewarned of this second description, and in reply to my question whether he had often thought of the illustrated cards of the last experiment, he usually replied that he had not thought about them at all." [1]

"The first decription presents the coexistence of the same two factors—impressional and emotional—which co-operated in the perception. According to the statements of the subjects, there remains in the eyes a certain trace, an internal vision, a mental copy, and sometimes a kind of feeling, a general impression, distinctly affective, upon which reproduction of the memory is founded."

"The second description is already the evocation of the image from the depths of the subconscious. It is, at the same time, the more or less distinct internal vision and memory of the preceding drawing and narration.

[1] Op. cit., p. 157.

One can even distinguish the part reproduced from the internal vision from the other part reproduced without the vision." They are two images. We may call them with Abramowski I_1 and I_2. In each of them we can discern the influence of intellectual activity.

Sometimes the first mental image approximates to a consecutive visual image when there is a trace of the impression remaining in the eye : it is thus a residue of perception. On the other hand, "cards perceived freely give rise to almost twice as many reproductions as those perceived with mental disturbance ; attention thus favours reproduction, distraction arising from interruptions is unfavourable to it." Likewise, the number of uncertainties appears to be proportional to the intensity of the factors of distraction and amnesia. In other terms, "intellectual inhibition of the perception diminishes the representative, intellectual part of the immediate image, increases its unconscious part, and at the same time brings this subconscious part nearer to the threshold of consciousness. On the contrary, the free activity of the intellect in perceptions increases the representative part of the image, diminishes its subconscious part and moves it away from the threshold of consciousness."[1]

The influence of intellectual activity on the subsequent mental image is still more manifest. This image is obtained a week after the first. It thus contains numerous elements : the subconscious difference between the perception and the first image, the difference between two images which have remained subconscious, the cryptamnesic history of the unconscious of the second degree and of the subconscious of the first degree.

In a general manner, this image is larger than the first. Here are a few figures. The increase taken on six different cards amounts from one series to the other to the following differences :—

[1] Op. cit., p. 179.

First Series.	Second Series.
0·18	0·73
0·22	0·30
0·58	0·67
0·21	0·34
0·20	0·19
0·56	0·40

Save in the case of the sixth card, and to a certain extent of the fifth, there is manifest progress from one series to the other, that is, subconscious creation.

According to Abramowski, these developments proceed from intellectual amnesia, the result of the interference of extraneous thoughts arising from study, distraction and from simultaneous amnesia and distraction accompanied by an emotion. The representative part of the image includes acquisitions of associative origin; the more numerous the associative paths the more the image is perfected.

On the other hand, if we consider the scale of subconscious creation in the case of individuals, we find it sensibly proportional to the degree of narrowness of consciousness and the extent of memory disturbed.

Finally, let us note the way the passage from the subconscious to the conscious is effected. The representative parts of the image are divided into two groups : the one " disappears during crytamnesia and pass into the subconscious, non-representative part of the memory ; the others, approaching the threshold, issue from the subconscious and reassume their intellectual aspect in augmenting the image."

Now these latent developments are in correlation with associations of affective origin. They are effected by a deviation of the attention in favour of an intense impression, by emotional interests, by the isolation of the emotional state, by what Freud calls " the imprisoned affectivity " ; what remains of the vision of images is a general impression which is rather affective, a kind of vague feeling.

In this form, the affective state is thus susceptible of a true fertility. This capacity is further reinforced by a crowd of actual dispositions. We have a sufficiently exact idea of this if we consider the effect of sensibility produced in us by the association of the concept of an object with the rich train of emotions which accompanied it in the past. A present, a portrait, a dried flower, a golden ring, the photograph of a religious ceremony, excite in our minds an eddy of feeling like that produced by a ship ploughing through the waves. We know that the verses of great poets awaken in readers their own emotions.

In the same way, in the scientific domain, accounts of the discoveries and inventions of others are able to produce a thrill of fertile exhilaration in the mind of the future scientist. In the courageous efforts of suffering genius to force its way upwards, the reader recognizes his own ordeal and strives towards a like end. It was not only Augustin Thierry who became aware of his vocation as an historian by reading Chateaubriand's *Martyrs* ; the life of the great builders of systems is full of these inward illuminations and bursts of enthusiasm following a piece of scientific reading, or the hearing of an inspiring lecture.

We may say with Ribot : " All forms of the creative imagination imply affective elements. This affective influence penetrates into the whole field of invention : for every invention pre-supposes an unsatisfied impulse, a state of gestation."

Further on the same author describes more exactly the way in which this co-operation of feeling and image takes place. He distinguishes two affective currents : the one constituting the emotion, the other inciting creation : " All affective dispositions can influence the creative imagination ; fear produces phantoms ; anger ruses in stratagem ; love creates an imaginary being substituted for the beloved object ; the creator has the pleasure of victory.[1]

[1] *L'imagination créatrice*, p. 26.

This is also doubtless the reason why, according to Bourdeau, spoken language is before all affective and pragmatic. "As a product of the unconscious reason, it expresses needs by expressing ideas and feelings."[1]

Why finally are ideas forces ? "It is," says Fouillée, "because they cover up appetites more or less vague. Ideas renew themselves by virtue of the bond uniting certain representations to certain feelings, and establishing in the brain certain reflex acts, certain paths of communication prepared for the reception of nerve currents. A dominating feeling or desire then finds paths by which it distributes itself and arouses suitable representations." In defining the rôle of the unconscious and the consciousness in the choice of concepts which are to be united, he adds : " Finally, consciousness becomes the principal source of the selection of ideas."

V. THE TRANSITION FROM THE UNCONSCIOUS TO CONSCIOUSNESS

We are thus brought, in a single step, to the conscious. This state is characterized, says Souriau, "by the surveillance of thoughts and images, the imposition of a programme determined by the mind, the intention. Ideas are cleared up and completed, the general plan of the work is elaboration. With the arrival of reflection the mind, forcing inspiration in a kind of way, enriches itself with new acquisitions and passes from the abstract to the concrete. If, with Bergson, we call the abstract idea " a pure virtuality containing the germ of all future development ", we may witht his penetrating philosopher sum up inventive work in the following words :—

" Intellectual work consists in conducting one and the same representation across different planes of

---

[1] Bourdeau, *La philosophie affective*, p. 31.

consciousness in a direction going from the abstract to the concrete, from the scheme to the image." [1]

This is not all. Taking into account the incessant reactions of feeling upon ideas, whether in the unconscious or the consciousness, we may complete the Bergsonian formula as follows : The entire work of the intellect conducts one and the same representation from the unconscious to the subconscious, from the subconscious to the consciousness, from the scheme to the image, from the abstract to the concrete, sometimes in the form of affective residues, sometimes in the form of intelligible concepts, sometimes under both of these aspects together.

VI. Summary and Conclusion

We have seen that feeling, being associated with idea in our conscious states, does not separate from the representative residues when the transition from consciousness to the unconscious is made.

But feeling does more. When this passage from clear and distinct states to mute and confused states takes place, the affective state succeeds to the representative state. There is thus conservation of psychical energy.

This emotional residue is associative, and governs the formation of judgments ; it is at one and the same time a static and dynamic energy. Thus it is active, and this activity is correlated with previous ideas which it inherits.

Being active, it is able to be fertile. Abramowski showed this ; Ribot and Fouillée recognized it. The image formed in the unconscious is the more developed, the more numerous have been associations of ideas previously conceived, the more it is in relationship with a rich affective state.

[1] Bergson, " L'effort intellectuel," in the *Revue philosophique*, 1902, vol. i, pp. 6, 11, 15, 16, 17. We may remark that Bergson regards the dynamic scheme as the simple representation capable of development into multiple images.

Thus in passing from the unconscious to the consciousness, a representation is carried from one state to another, from a simple form to a complex form, from the affective state to the intelligible state, from the abstract state to the concrete state, from the embryonic state of a fertile idea to the developed state of an invention.

We have seen how this analysis is verified in the history of scientific inventions, at the origin of which we have always found a strong desire or need, or a passion for discovery.

In the case of all great constructors, we find this affective memory penetratingly analysed by Paulhan, which, in a state of unceasing evolution, and reinforced by other memories or increased by new acquisitions, becomes the bond of union between unconscious and conscious states.

From this we see the importance of the æsthetic unconscious. The automatic unconscious alone is a reservoir of psychical residues. Being associated with the dynamic unconscious, it has developed this hidden reserve. But neither one nor the other could be fertile without the aid of feeling, each form of which is original, and, as the ferment of life and expansion, is found at the beginning of all inventions.

The soul in quest of new things is not a cold mind. Whether its researches are effected in the full light of consciousness, or whether they are silently elaborated in the mysterious zones of the lower psychism, they are always active and directed by invisible tendencies, by desires, by needs, by a whole gamut of feeling which appears to be latent, until it bursts forth in the joyous enthusiasm of discovery.

This indissoluble alliance between mind and heart in the glorious conquest of thought has been celebrated in excellent terms by an artist, the painter Albert Besnard :—

" Intelligence and passion are very close to genius. Who in our century will have the honour of bringing them together ? We cannot yet know, the struggle blinds us, but posterity will pronounce the verdict." [1]

We may reassure the eloquent Academician. This combination of which he dreams has existed in all civilized nations. The Apostles of scientific progress went to seek truth " with all their soul " as Plato would have them. Feeling has always cleared the way for the idea. We have just proved this by analysis. The following chapter will bring the final confirmation. In a study of the synthesis of inventive work effected by virtue of the unconscious it will show for the last time the interpenetration of the various forms of psychical force in scientific inventions.

[1] Discourse by M. L. Barthou, in reply to a discourse by M. A. Besnard, at the Academie francaise, 10th June, 1926.

CHAPTER V

SYNTHESIS OF THE WORK ACCOMPLISHED BY THE UNCONSCIOUS IN SCIENTIFIC INVENTION

The unconscious is above all automatic in the preparation of the invention—the unconscious is above all dynamic in the conception of the invention—the unconscious is both dynamic and æsthetic in the development and modification of the invention—the unconscious is at once automatic, dynamic, and æsthetic in the verification of the invention—summary.

OUR analysis has shown us the unconscious, whether in the form of psychical results preserved in automatism, or in the effects of a hidden dynamism, or finally, in the transformative influence of an affective state. We have now to solve the following question :—

How does the unconscious act at each of these phases ? Under what form is it effective ? In the necessary interpenetration of feeling, ideas, and activity, how does the unconscious manifest itself as the organizer of scientific invention ? To sum up, it is the synthesis of inventive work which we are endeavouring to reconstitute. We shall have brought into relief the rôle of the various conscious or subconscious factors when we have considered them in turn in the preparation of invention, in the conception of the hypothesis, in the development and transformation of the directing idea, and finally in the verification of the invention.

I. THE UNCONSCIOUS IN THE PREPARATION OF THE INVENTION

At the beginning, the mind has only certain predispositions in one direction or the other of research. It is thus the hereditary unconscious which gives to future inventors the initial direction of their studies. They make observations by instinct, in a direction indicated by nature. The unconscious is at its lowest degree in their sensibility, in their sensibility without memory; they experience sensorial impressions which are not linked together, vague feelings; these are "the conscious product of an unconscious valuation".

But inventing is combining. On the other hand, these combinations will be the more numerous and varied the richer the capital of material accumulated in the mind. We thus see the future genius in quest of innumerable elements for synthesis. Watt and George Stevenson are never tired of examining and constructing models; Pasteur studies crystals, as revealing the admirable order of nature; Cuvier studies the peculiarities of the bones of animals; Darwin the instincts of honey bees. Furthermore, this acquisition is favoured by good health, by a cheerful temperament, and by physical energy. Some find a momentary excess of energy in stimulants, such as coffee and alcohol; all are concerned with facilitating the work of their imagination without injury to that of their memory; in all cases, this memory is remarkable; in the cases of Cuvier, Ampère and Poincaré it is extraordinary.

They read a great deal, and without thinking about it, link the ideas of others with their own personal conceptions —which itself is already invention—and in making this unconscious combination, they prepare the way for original thoughts: Galilei reads Euclid, Cuvier is inspired by Buffon, and the naturalist Bonnet studies a work of Réaumur.

Not content with learning, they write essays and these compositions force them to round off and precisify their ideas which are thus as it were "held in leash"; they exchange their conceptions with others and this expression modifies and enriches their thoughts: "Language," says Souriau, "is a form of invention." [1] We may even say with him "that it is a thinking machine".

[1] Souriau, *Théorie de l'invention*, p. 127.

Then, in the first years of adolescence, we have the beginnings of experiment : Watt fits up and dismantles tools ; Wurtz, the future chemist, experiments with furnaces of brick in the washhouse ; Ampère does mathematics with small pebbles. In all these attempts, they are obeying an instinctive tendency, a true unconscious logic.[1] They were to know later, with proof to support them, that many causes can produce the same effect ; and they are not ignorant that certain causes depend upon one another, and that others, when in association, may sometimes reinforce and sometimes oppose one another. But, long before their inventions, they suspect this interdependence, intersubstitution, and interference of causes. That is why, driven by the desire for discovery, they enlarge the frame of their knowledge. Pasteur takes lessons in zoology from H. Fabre, because, being only a chemist, he has a vague desire to become a microbiologist ; Ampère, who shone as a physicist, began with poetry and mathematics, continued with chemistry and biology, and, during the whole of his life, had a passion for metaphysics.

Being one day called upon to effect truly revolutionary changes, they reveal the traces which recall the past to them, because these traces, as precious relics, allow them to construct their future syntheses through analogy and hypothesis. They realize that the principle of the constancy of the laws of nature is not sufficient to prove that the stone, for example, will always fall in the same manner ; they take account of the factor of time, that is to say, the history of the past. Who knows, they say to themselves, whether nature, like man, has not also " its epochs, that is to say, laws in which time plays an essential part " ? That is why, says Cournot, " they attribute great importance to the data of history." [2]

In this way a great mass of material is accumulated for

[1] Loridan, *Nos savants*, pp. 38, 39.
[2] Cournot, *Traité de l'enchainement des idées fondamentales dans les sciences et dans l'histoire*, Paris, 1911, p. 207.

further construction. But in this multiplicity of observations, in this progressive enrichment of memory, in these numerous associations of images and ideas, we have discovered the unconscious : it is found on the threshold of perception ; it appears in the cause of the revival of memories ; it is in the general idea, as a point of departure for associations and in the feeling which inspires secondary ideas ; it is necessary to the formation and combination of images ; finally, we find it in intellectual assimilation, the prelude to mental synthesis, and at the beginnings of judgment and reasoning.

Nevertheless, so far the unconscious is not essentially dynamic and æsthetic, although it governs activity and is vaguely present in the elaboration of thought. It registers the results attained ; it conserves mental acquisitions ; in the division of labour of the operations of the spirit, it represents the employee who keeps the books and presides over the ledger. But it is not the director whose initiative provides for the development of enterprises. The preparation of the scientific invention is thus effected principally by the automatic unconscious.

II. The Unconscious in the Conception of the Invention

In the reaction of the mind upon the elements contained in it, certain combinations are formed. These are, first of all, those which are possible we may here survey, with Tarde, the infinite army of possibilities. These are conditional certainties, since, when certain conditions are realized, they will come into existence. They are conceived by observation of the connection of facts. Their like reproduction in analogous circumstances allows us to assert other facts for other circumstances not yet observed.[1] Thus, above life and the flux of realities, there is a network of possibilities. When a new element of this whole complex is realized the infinite mass of

[1] Tarde, *Logique sociale*, p. 154.

conditional certainties advances one degree towards existence.

But this passage from possibilities to existence implies the realization of certain conditions. Tarde sums these up in the words : " The point of maturity of possibilities."

This maturity may be conceived objectively and subjectively.

Objectively, it expresses the state of science which allows a certain discovery or invention to be borne. Accurately speaking, it is a fundamental discovery which renders possible further discoveries and inventions derived from the first. We have found plenty of examples of this. But, from the subjective point of view, the problem must be stated differently. Why is a certain possibility realized rather than another ? Why are B and C excluded ?˙ It is because A, B and C are not presented alone to the eye of the mind as concepts. Like the charming theory of the young girls between whom Ahasuerus had to make his choice, the ideas A, B and C show themselves with all the variety of their attractions and in all the grades of their beauties. Each is accompanied by a train of affective phenomena which give it value. For, on the one hand, the intellectual tendencies cause joy or pain. On the other hand, the invention which is in course of preparation is a new phenomenon, and thus not associated with others. Finally, the inventions inspired by desires are attached to passions. The result of this is an affective disturbance, a pleasure or a pain. The causes of this complex emotive state are numerous. Generally, it is the systematization of ideas, a labour which may be agreeable or painful ; surprise arising from the new thing glimpsed ; weariness of seeing a system built up slowly, or the joy of seeing it finished at last ; sometimes, it is an unsatisfied passion which expends itself in intellectual invention ; in this case the invention, an ideal satisfaction, is substituted for the real satisfaction. The scientific hypothesis will assuage a desire, as a novel works a love. Under the evocative influence of this emotion, a selection is effected first of all in the feelings, and then in the ideas. *A* is preferred to *B* and *C* because it is supported by a sounder affective group. There is a choice, and hence the rejection of certain elements and the union of others. We have, says Tarde, destructive criticism followed by inventive creation. It is the logical duel followed by the logical union. Consequently, every development produces the destruction of parallel beginnings; at every move forward towards a precise realization, the mind has to sacrifice latent aptitudes.[1]

But how has the new system, reduced to its essential idea, been formed ? On the one hand, the invention is a real acquisition for the mind. On the other hand, reasoning only brings forward identical ideas, and never a new concept. In geometry, says Souriau, it is not *B* that is contained in *A*, it is *A* which is found in *B* together with other things. Geometry is not therefore deducted but invented. Thus logic makes reasoning comprehensible but does not construct it.

On the other hand, the imagination combines, but does not create in the true sense. It is therefore necessary to pass beyond imagination in order to produce the birth of the fertile idea.

Must we stop at reflection ? It limits reverie; it fixes our mind on an abstract idea, it causes other ideas to rise up which are connected with those under consideration. But too much reflection is injurious; minds which are too reflective are short-sighted; we need to leave minds a certain amount of liberty in order that they may see far and high, for digressions are useful. Invention is thus not the intentional work of the mind.[2]

It is certainly the work of chance, as Souriau thinks, but let us define in what sense this is true. " Chance, writes this psychologist, " is the conflict between external

---

[1] Paulhan, *Psychologie de l'invention*, pp. 28, 40, 41. Tarde : *Logique sociale*, pp. 172–200.

[2] Souriau, op. cit., p. 24.

causality and internal finality." There is no chance
outside ourselves. In one way or another, everything
is determined. On the other hand, there is no chance
in ourselves, since our will is determined in some way
by the acts which precede it and is determinant with
regard to those which follow it. But there is chance
in the interference between the series of external
phenomena, which are strangers to the ego, and the
series of internal phenomena which depend upon the
ego. Thus chance becomes the unforeseen. It is not a
negation of cause, it is the unexpected but nevertheless
real cause, the unconscious cause. When the Rhone
disappears into its subterranean bed at Bellegarde, to
reappear later, it is not its course which is discontinuous,
it is the external manifestation of this cause. The same
is true of fortuitous causes.

The discontinuity is in the consciousness ; continuity
exists in the logical connection between the antecedents
and the consequence. That is why chance only exists
for an imperfect intelligence. In the eye of a mind which,
like God, would see the total interconnection of the
phenomena of the Universe in their whole synthesis,
there would be no such thing as chance.

Hence, the invention is not determined in its totality
either by the concepts already acquired, nor by the
suggestions coming from the external world. It results
from the interference of these two currents. Is this
saying enough ? Our previous analysis has taught us
how acquisitions from outside modify unceasingly the
concepts of the mind, how these are constantly influenced
by sensibility and will, how the unconscious residues
of our whole past find their echo in the least of our
actual thoughts. We may draw this conclusion, that the
governing idea, the mother of the invention, is in a
direction determined by previous preparation and native
tendencies, the final result of these partly conscious
and partly unconscious transformations.

We thus have the hypothesis, which was a mild light

for Newton, a sudden brilliance for Archimedes and Poincaré. It is the anticipation of the law ; it is the directing idea for future construction ; it is the theory conceived before being established ; it is the flight of the mind which, by the use of its wings, reaches summits to which no path leads ; it is, says Liebig, " the thought which precedes the experiment." The unconscious causes it to be born in various ways : in the affective state which presided over the decisive choice ; in the general analogy which inspired a certain derived idea ; in the imagination which fuses together into a whole several images without our being able to account for this fusion ; in the driving idea, the basis of assimilation and prelude to mental synthesis ; in the judgment of identification which constitutes the hypothesis itself, that is to say, in the mental state regarded before its apperception by the mind.

In this mysterious force which effects selections and syntheses, there is more than automatism, a purely static unconscious ; there is no predominance of the æsthetic unconscious, since, if feeling accompanied the invisible elaboration, it did not inspire a final form of the invention, since the hypothesis is capable of revision. When we reduce it to the correct propositions of a directive thought full of virtualities, and of an embryo capable of many transformations, the invention is above all the product of the dynamic unconscious.

III. The Unconscious in the Development and Modification of the Invention

The fundamental idea of the invention has been conceived. It encloses a world of possibilities. How is it going to develop ?

Exactly like an ordinary thought, the simplest that we can imagine, for every thought with its original physiognomy is an invention. Let us take this subject for development. Life is a battle. An elementary analysis shows me a triple life and hence a triple field of battle : the life of the body, hence the combat of the body ; life of the intelligence, and hence conflicts of thought ; the moral life, and hence the struggles of will and heart. But at the same time I determine the elements of this analysis, I extended the subject to a diversity of objects ; the subject has behaved like a drop of oil ; its development has been at once a deepening by analysis and a widening by the synthesis of objects which I have attached to the fundamental idea. In this double progress of my thought, the essential points of the analysis alone have been found by the conscious efforts of logic. The images and recollections which were evoked appeared in order to support the directing idea, as a result of an unconscious suggestion ; in short, the development of every thought implies a comprehensive analysis of its contents and an extensive synthesis of the secondary ideas which it annexes.

The first operation is not properly called an invention ; it does not cause anything new to be seen, but it causes us to see more clearly ; it is at most a progress in clarity. The second operation is the essential element of the invention ; it is a conquest, an annexation. The whole development will be nothing but a series of new annexations, a sheaf of conquests effected by the unconscious and organized by conscious logic. These two ideas— progressive annexations and synthetic organization— describe the whole process of the development of the invention.

But precisely by reason of this victorious character of the directing idea, secondary ideas attach themselves to the first.

It is impossible to divine *a priori* their number and their relative dynamism. On the other hand, the bond which unites them to the initial hypothesis will be more or less direct and, in so far, will determine within the collection of ideas, a more or less strong bond between the constituting parts and the whole so constituted.

Paulhan bases upon this diversity of importance and cohesion his distinction between the development of the invention by evolution, by transformation, and by deviation.

The point of departure of the first procedure is a general principle. This principle is a germ. Secondary ideas are derived from the first, either by unconscious inspiration or by more or less conscious reasoning. In this case the consciousness only comes in at a certain degree of organization : " Unconscious genius," says Paulhan, " is found more or less in the case of all inventors, and a part of the invention always remains unconscious for one reason or another, whether because it is not sufficiently closely attached to the ego or because it is too closely attached. In the evolution of an invention there are always many elements which are neither will nor felt. But in certain cases, the unconscious becomes general." [1]

Altogether, in the case of this procedure, the system is closely linked together. Evolution has been normal with phases of consciousness and unconsciousness.

Altogether different is the development by transformation. In this case one element, endowed with a stronger affective dynamism, becomes predominant ; it soon stifles the principal and replaces it. Later on, a series of evolutions will follow one another in the same fashion and the transformation will never be complete. Thus, the bond of the system has been relaxed ; the initial tendency has, however, subsisted ; but a new work has been formed around the principal idea ; new elements have transformed it without the knowledge of the inventor ; a stable element has remained, but the initial development has been continued in an altered sense.

Transformation of the invention changes the orientation, but the work remains single. In development by deviation, two works are developed in parallel with one another. In consequence of a very lively impression, of the

[1] Paulhan, *Psychologie de l'invention*, p. 97.

awakening of a powerful feeling, of the intricate tendencies of an original mind, of the addition to the original system of syntheses of images coming from the totality of our state of consciousness, of an attempt at correction of original work, one creation separates from the other, and generally develops at its expense. If the mind is supple and vigorous, this duplication is the source of great fertility. But most often, one of the psychical germs dies while the other grows. As in the case of transformation, deviation thus produces the death of ideas : these germs coming into being in a mind too weak to allow them to flourish and fructify, have not been viable. Sometimes, however, they may reappear, rescued by the unconscious which attaches them to a new synthesis. The latter will thus be composed of unexpected elements. It will be one of those hybrid products which defy all analysis, but a product which is perhaps formed very frequently. Who knows out of what debris collected unconsciously by mental synthesis our ordinary judgments, our ingenious little notions, our most simple as well as our boldest psychical combinations, are made ?

To sum up, as Paulhan says, invention is always systematization, a crystalization of the thought around a primitive nucleus. It is a series of little inventions similar to the one first conceived ; if they are all assimilated to the first, there is evolution ; if they separate from it, we have transformation or deviation as the case may be.

All the same, this distinction between the three procedures of development, however ingenious it may be, is more apparent than real. As regards the rôle of the unconscious in it, the process is fundamentally identical in the three cases. We can easily prove this if we compare modifications of the hypothesis, or of the initial invention, in the case of most inventors.

Do we really find in some cases pure logical evolution, in others simple transformation, and in others again deviation properly so called ?   Do we not have in all cases at once persistence of a constant and primitive element, and thus evolution, and variation by the addition of heterogenous elements, and thus transformation and deviation ?

In order to settle this question, we may refer again to a few of the facts which have formed the subject of our inquiry, chosen from each of the categories of scientific invention.

Leibniz starts out from his metaphysical theory of universal continuity ; he reads the " indivisibles " of Cavalieri, the mitre of Pascal, the quadratures and rectification of curves by Fermat ; he finds the principles of the differential calculus in Fermat and those of the integral calculus in Pascal ; he accepts these principles ; he generalizes the special solutions and creates the language—itself another generalization of the infinitesimal calculus.   In this development there is certainly evolution of the one and the same principle, but also the unconscious annexation of diverse elements which prolong and complete it.

Laplace, for his part, proceeded by successive extensions. He started from the theory of Buffon on the common origin of planets and satellites ; this was the hypothesis in its first stage ; he modified it according to certain observations on the uniform sense of planetary motions, on the smallness of the eccentricity of the orbits of comets, on the existence of the rings of Saturn.   In endeavouring to account for these observed facts, he explained by the conception of his nebular hypothesis, not only the formation of the sun, but also that of planets, satellites, and comets.   The primitive hypothesis was enlarged ; its development was a series of annexations ; thanks to the unconscious process, there was continuity of the initial principles and diversity in its extension.

The same work of amplification is found again in the case of Newton.   He sees the apple fall and the flash of identification shines in his eyes.   His hypothesis was not changed in nature from its initial form, but was enriched with new elements.

The same observation can be made concerning the inventions in physical science most often made in collaboration. Torricelli glimpsed the existence of the atmospheric pressure. Pascal gave the general law of it. We have at once permanence of the same principle and very varied extension of it. Oerstedt carried out his experiments ; Ampère and Arago generalized the range of them : telegraphy is the result of this extension. Niepce discovered the property of asphaltum ; Daguerre discovered the developer ; both, starting out from the hypothesis that light can be fixed, realized photography by completing their directing idea by a secondary idea which prolonged it.

Claude Bernard carried out a series of experiments based upon the hypothesis that the body manufactured sugar, and in showing that the seat of this manufacture was the liver the original idea was only made more precise and not weakened. Pasteur's hypothesis of immunization, once found by chance, was diversified in its application, but always came back to this formula : immunize in order to heal.

This conquering power of the directing idea is not less great in the moral sciences.

Before finding his laws of *imitation*, Tarde made an hypothesis concerning universal difference and finished with a theory of universal similarity, a manifest deviation, it will be said. This is apparently the case, but not so fundamentally. For if experience modified the expression of his first hypothesis, there exists between the two a common element. In the same way that black and white, so opposite to one another, belong to the same genus colour, in the same way difference and resemblance are of the same genus quality. This is true of all contraries. Association by contrast may be assimilated, as we have observed, to association by resemblance. Thus the same logical evolution caused the author to pass from his first hypothesis to the second ; we always find a certain identity under diversity.

Descartes offers us a similar example in philosophy. The " admirable science " of which he dreamed reduces to three principles : (1) In order to arrive at certitude, we must start from the ego ; (2) Certitude is a truth of intuition ; (3) Divine veracity is the guarantee of knowledge. These are three forms of the hypothesis. One implies the other : God is perfect, hence he does not wish to deceive the philosopher in what his reason tells him ; hence His existence, a fact of intuition, is a certainty. It is easy to see the unity underlying this three-fold expression of the foundation of human knowledge.

Even Auguste Comte offers us a coherent system, in spite of the two opposed forms in which his philosophy is clothed. His relation with Clotilde de Vaux formed the occasion for his introducing feeling into his philosophy ; after the primacy of positive reason, the primacy of the heart. An aberration on the part of the master, said Littré indignantly. A fine example of deviation, Paulhan will say. Neither one nor the other, in our opinion. As Picard says, whom we have already quoted, logical continuity exists between the positive doctrine of the *Three States*, and the discourse which introduced the *Religion of Humanity* ; but we shall supply a different reason from his. Comte sums up thus his social thesis : *Love* as principle, *Order* as basis, and *Progress* as goal. Now in his theory of the Three States he already pursues progress by means of order. He has thus not changed as regards order and progress. He has simply substituted love for the synthesis operated by positive reason in the first plan. But this is precisely because, according to him, " Love effects the social synthesis as logic effects the positive synthesis." He has thus progressed, starting from the same basis, *order*, towards the same goal, *progress*, by grafting on the first system a new element, which· is the true effective link, *love*. We have thus a continuity of the same principle but variation in the secondary ideas derived from it.[1]

Finally, in technology, we may take the case of Gutenberg. His hypothesis developed in three successive leaps : The apparatus had to reproduce a picture, it had to be a press, it had to reproduce letters like a die. The fundamental idea reappears in each development. He wished " to simplify the work of the copyists ". We must always find the unity of the original hypothesis under the diversity of successive realization. In the case of George Stevenson, the machines invented before the " Rocket " each represent a partial invention before the final invention ; we thus have progress, but continuity of the directing idea, and each time the addition of new elements which form part of the final whole.

Thus, in all these developments, we find again the essential element of the primordial hypothesis. Now this evolution has taken place, as we have seen, by means of the association of ideas, of imagination, of analogy, of intuition and of reasoning. On the other hand, we know all the phases of unconsciousness which must be interpolated into the course of these intellectual operations. Furthermore, we have shown the considerable place occupied by sensibility in this creative process, the ardent desire, passion for discovery, or sometimes simply the need of perfecting unfinished inventions.

Consequently, logical continuity requires the concurrence of both the dynamic unconscious and the æsthetic unconscious in order to effect the connection between the original form of the invention and the complicated machinery of its development ; this unconscious is necessary, since conscious reason cannot take account of the various stages of this evolution, the logical character of which, however, it recognizes after the final construction. This unconscious is dynamic, since the inventor, using the attempts of his predecessors,

[1] These two conceptions of Comte originated in Saint Simon. Cf. Segond, in *Revue de Synthèse historique*, vol. xv, of the new series.

reading and observation, has brought about the growth of the primitive theme ; this unconscious is æsthetic, since as the heir of intellectual forces the consciousness of which has disappeared, it directs tendencies towards the goal to be reached and because, being naturally associated, it harmonizes and fuses into coherent groups the elements developed.

Nevertheless, the rôle of this invisible agent is not terminated. We find it at the side of logical reason in the verification of the invention.

IV. The Unconscious in the Verification of the Invention

First of all, we do not need to seek the influence of the unconscious in certain intellectual operations which are needed, it is true to verify invention, but are clearly followed by the eye of the mind. In fact, the full light of consciousness bears upon the judgment of perception, the conclusion of reasoning, the calculations made by Laplace, Ampère and Poincaré to test the results of their intuitions, the experiments made by Torricelli, Pascal, Ampère, Malus, Claude Bernard, to force Nature to reveal clearly the secrets of her laws. The attempts made by the constructors of machines before the realization of the final apparatus, and finally, the correction of the first hypothesis according to the result of calculation.

But this mysterious action reappears in verification for two reasons : (1) Because this control requires intellectual operations, which, according to our analysis, contain an element of unconsciousness. (2) Because the experimental sciences imply a succession of experiments suggested one by another. Now this process of evocation, as we have seen, has its unconscious aspects.

To control is to prove, either by reasoning or by experiment. Now reasoning includes the recollections of memory, the mental images of the imagination, and the analogies of judgment. But we have already marked off the zone occupied by the unconscious in the operations.

On the other hand, experiment is long and varied. As conducted by Pasteur, Claude Bernard, and Ampère, it is, as we have seen, a series of attempts each conditioning the next; for example, a detail observed is recorded in the experiment C_1; without it being thought about it will enter into the judgment which renders necessary, for the sake of completeness, the experiment C_2. This, in its turn, is judged to be insufficient; nevertheless, certain observed details have struck the experimentor; later on, without his accounting to himself exactly for this relation, he will try the experiment C_3, which will make use of details previously found in order to become the conclusive experiment.

Finally, if we reduce reasoning to a series of experiments in thought—while maintaining reservations with regard to this theory of Rignano—all the intellectual operations of our mind, like all our external experiences, becomes series of judgments implied one by the other, called up one by the other, or completed one by the other, until we arrive at the final mental synthesis which decides the result.

V. SUMMARY

We may now sum up the work accomplished, when the experiments are finished, the calculations completed, and verifications achieved. The preparation of the invention was long, sometimes conscious and sometimes unconscious; in its obscure phases, it utilizes above all the automatic unconscious. The birth of the invention takes place sometimes by a sudden flash, sometimes by slow crystallization, and it is then elaborated principally by the dynamic unconscious. The development and modification of the invention, with their phases of intuition, reasoning, and fresh intuition, are the joint work of the dynamic unconscious effecting annexations and the æsthetic unconscious unifying the results. Finally, in the verification of the hypothesis, automatism has recorded the last observations, the dynamic unconscious suggests the ultimate development, and the æsthetic unconscious directs the whole process of reasoning towards the final invention.

GENERAL CONCLUSIONS

TO conclude this study, we may draw two kinds of conclusions : The one relating to the inventor, the other to the invention itself regarded as part of science.

I. RELATING TO THE INVENTOR

(a) There is not more in the human mind than in the external world. There is no spontaneous generation. The invention is thus prepared for at length : Previous study organizes automatism and formulates groups of thoughts into summarized insight. The future constructor accumulates as much material as possible ; he directs it, he lives in it ; he thinks it over again in his own way and translates the ideas of others ; he prepares himself for psychological unity by great efforts of analysis and synthesis. Always alert, " his mind," writes Le Roy, "is in a state of continual vibration like the antennae of certain insects." Its acquisitions reinforce one another ; preserved in the automatic unconscious, developed by the dynamic unconscious, canalized by the aesthetic unconscious. They effect, by becoming the total unconscious, the progressive maturation of thought.

(b) In this way, the unconscious economizes spiritual power. The progress is accomplished in the mind without the intervention of consciousness ; in a sense, as in external nature, nothing is lost, everything is transformed. This conservation of psychical energy causes intellectual representations to pass to the affective state in order that they may be suddenly revived one day, after unconscious elaboration, in the form of an original idea, a bold thought which appears in consciousness before rational control : This is the hypothesis. This product is the result of a preliminary dissociation of the psychical elements followed by a new association. The more the mind is capable of this dissolution of pre-existing syntheses, the more fertile it is in inventions.

(c) Through the agency of the reconstructive work of the unconscious, a double intuition is produced : the *initial* intuition of the hypothesis, and the *final* intuition of the value of the reasoning. These two intuitions are syntheses, the one vague and confused, the other clear and distinct. The various modalities of reasoning link together the details of conscious analysis. The method followed by the inventive scientist is thus neither a sequence of syntheses, nor a sequence of analyses; it is a long analysis between two syntheses, a long process of reasoning between two intuitions. In this process, intuition furnishes all the points of departure, discursive dialectic prolongs them and verifies them. This is the circular method, the true and only scientific method.

(d) The unconscious reappears in various degrees in all mental operations which combine in invention, even in judgment and in reasoning.

The divination of an analogy is thus not explained, as Desdouits thought, by simple habit of mind : " The latter, he says, leaps over the intermediaries to the conclusion." For these intermediaries exist, nevertheless, in unconscious activity. We agree with him in saying that every judgment is an assertion, but he assumes consciousness, either of certainty or doubt. But we add : this assertion is not an assertion without an object; it is the assertion of an entity, although here of an unconscious mental state which precedes the assertion of which it is the expression.

(e) Passing to the invention itself, we agree with Joyau in seeing in it a work of logic. The creative imagination aids the reason in drawing all the conclusions from a principle ; it constructs them, and, to this extent,

Y

as Goblot says, scientific deduction goes beyond the limits of the syllogism properly so called. But Joyau mistakes the rôle of chance and external phenomena as they affect the mind of the inventor when he writes : "In inspiration, the human mind is essentially progressive ; if it advances, it is by virtue of its own energy and not by external influences ; the objects which surround it, the phenomena and forces which act upon it, far from assisting and favouring development, can only deflect it or arrest it." [1]

(*f*) Finally, in various degrees, we have shown the unconscious and subconscious in the evolution of ideas, in the formation of affective states, in the preparation of the invention, in its development, and, partly, in its verification. The sum total of the psychical operations which collaborate in the invention forms a continuous series in which we can distinguish conscious and unconscious phases. Hence, if we follow Dupont in representing O_1, O_2, O_3 . . . the objective chain complete and continuous, by C_1, C_2, C_3 . . . . the facts which have a conscious manifestation by P_1, P_2, P_3 . . . . the facts which have a phenomenal manifestation, we have the following table showing the complete psychical process of the operation of invention :—

$$\ldots\ldots\ldots C_1 - C_2 - C_3 - C_4 - C_5 - C_6 - C_7 \ldots\ldots\ldots\ldots$$
$$O_1 - O_2 - O_3 - O_4 - O_5 - O_6 - O_7 - O_8 - O_9 - O_{10} - O_{11} - O_{12}$$
$$P_1 - P_2 - P_3 - P_4 - P_5 \ldots\ldots P_6 - P_7 - P_8 \ldots\ldots$$

This scheme shows us, in the series O_1, O_2, etc. ; all the factors utilized in scientific creation. We also see that among these facts some have both a phenomenal manifestation P, and a conscious manifestation C, others a phenomenal manifestation P alone, others,

---

[1] Joyau, *De l'invention dans les arts, dans les sciences et dans la pratique de la vertue*, pp. xii, xiii.

finally, a conscious manifestation C without phenomenal manifestation. If we complete this representation by the special formulæ which we have given in the theory of integral knowledge with reference to the discontinuity of consciousness in the operation of reasoning, we obtain the symbolic summary of the psychology of the rôle of the unconscious in invention.[1]

II. WITH REGARD TO THE INVENTION CONSIDERED AS A PART OF SCIENCE.

" The aim of the scientist ", says Le Roy, " is the progress and convergence of thought. Philosophy is the spirit of invention conscious of its steps, the spirit of reflective invention ; it seeks the principle of progress in the verification and realization of being."

Nothing could be more exact ; this movement of the mind is essentially a conquering march. Consequently, in science, the point of view of *position, productivity, genesis,* is more important than the point of view of *result.*

At the beginning, the mind sets forth in mystery. In fact, as we have seen, too much rigour and precision paralyse invention : " Every system, says Boutroux, is factitious ; it excludes all nuances. Too much cohesion is the mark of artificiality ; contradictions are factitious, says Le Roy ; they cling to words ; reality is not contradictory, but in course of resolution. Conquently, the inventor leaves the discursive surface of the mind for its supra-logical depths. His logic is rather a metaphysics. Invention is the passage from one plane of thought to another, hence the reversal of customary thought, a true conversion." [2]

However, we do not think, as does Le Roy, that invention is effected in the realm of contradiction, nor

[1] Dupont, *Les problèmes de la philosophie et leur enchainement scientifique* p. 314.
[2] Le Roy, *Revue de metaphysique et de morale,* 1905, pp. 193–223.

that the spirit of invention "assumes belief in the evolution of evidence, and the plasticity of reason". Logical evidence, considered in itself, does not change. Reason, for its part, is not modified by the fact of an invention. An element previously unknown has entered into a combination to form a new system ; we are thus obliged, while supported by the first principles, to accept this new synthesis in the same way that, previously and supported by the same principles, we accepted another. What has been changed is not the rational foundation of our judgments, but the matter of these judgments.

For, as Le Roy recognizes, the invention is a synthesis, and thus a work of logic.

Consequently, the scientific inventor is more than a constructor, he is a critic. " His invention is tested first of all, that is to say, verified. Thus, it is no longer something Utopian, it bears two signs of truth : Experience and duration."

On the other hand, the greater part of inventions, above all in the domain of physics, are effected in collaboration. Preparation is thus collective, achievement is individual ; the differentiating element which each carries within himself is the principle of the originality of the work. Every creative mind becomes a kind of wave on the social river, similar to others in certain aspects, but distinguished from them by its own form and prolonging the actions of the others. Thus the sum total of the conquest of science is effected at once by individuals and by society. It marches towards a unity which Hannequin has characterized as follows :—

" Science and philosophy only separate in order to be able to better penetrate the mystery of the real and to recover the unity of the effort which creates them and of the knowledge which is their common aim ; the progress of any particular science reacts upon that of all the others. Science lives by a variety of theories which agree with one another in a superior unity. The spirit of initiative and invention is formed by contact with present or passed inventions." [1]

Thus, if we consider it in its totality, the development of science results at once from the continuity of the initial principle and from gradual extensions of this principle. Hence, the inventor, who is enriched with abundant recollections and groups them easily in new constructions, is the pioneer of universal order. " That is why, says Goblot, invention seems to be the most eminent of intellectual qualities. An intelligent man finds that of which others have no notion." In fact, the uninterrupted succession of inventions is the progressive revelation of order. For the true is order conceived ; the good order desired ; the beautiful order felt. Now we know that in this vast universe, gaps have been noticed, unknown things have been perceived. Inventors immediately set to work. They have faith in final causes ; and, because invention implies discovery and creation, they unite scientific curiosity with artistic taste, the love of science with the passion for beauty. Now, says Maeterlinck, the moment when an object appears to us most admirable is that in which we have the best opportunity for perceiving its truth. The beauty which we lend to it directs our attention to its real beauty and grandeur which are not easy to discover and consist in the relations which every object necessarily has with the general and eternal laws and forces. [2]

Such is the secret of the joy of scientific conquerors, of the enthusiasm of Archimedes, of the admiring ecstasy of Kepler and Newton in face of the beauty of the laws which they discovered. The truths which they pursue are like stars seen separately in the sky. Glory to those who discover one of these golden stars in the firmament of science, sometimes without knowing what they do, and sometimes armed with a telescope.

[1] Hannequin, *Étude d'histoire des sciences et d'histoire de la philosophie*, Paris, 1908, pp. 22–40.

[2] Quoted by Boucaud, *Esquisse de l'ordre universel*, Paris, 1925, p. 62.

They realize genius and create beauty, because they have in their hearts the sacred flame of desire ; they reach the light and find as it were a sketch of the universal order. They become poets in every sense of the word : Because, while the Saints, as Janet says, are the " poets of the Good " the inventors in the domain of science are the poets of the True.

BIBLIOGRAPHY

ABRAMOWSKI (EDOUARD). *Le subconscient normal*, Paris, 1914.
Quoted with reference to the relations between the image and the recollection.

ANTOINE (E.). *La vie et les oeuvres de Pierre Laffite*, Le Havre, 1881.
Information concerning Comte's positivism.

ARISTOTLE. *De anima*, book iii, chap. v.
He speaks of a certain subconscious activity.
[Greek, with English translation, introduction, and notes by R. D. Hicks.]

ASLAN. *Expérience et invention en morale*, Paris, 1908.
The author expounds the formation of a theoretical system of morals.

AUGUSTINE (SAINT). *Confessions*, vol. x.
We find there a theory of the psychological unconscious.
[Numerous English translations.]

BACON (FRANCIS). *Novum Organum*, i; *De interpretatione naturae*, vol. iii; *De augmentis scientiarum*, vol. v.
Quoted in connection with scientific invention.

BAIN (ALEXANDER). *The Senses and the Intellect*, London, 1855.
The rôle of emotion in invention.

BARTHELEMY (SAINT-HILAIRE.) *Philosophie des deux Ampère*, Paris, 1966.
The author expounds in particular the theory of relations of Andre-Marie Ampère.

BELLET (DANIEL). *Dernières inventions, dernières decouvertes*, Paris, 1921.

BERGSON. *Creative Evolution*, translated by Mitchell, London, 1911.
Matter and Memory, translated by Paul and Palmer, London, 1911. " L'effort intellectuel," *Revue philosophique*, 1902, vol. i.
"Introduction à la métaphysique," *Revue de métaphysique*, 1903. Referred to in connection with the theory of intuition, and in regard to intellectual work, conscious and unconscious in turn.
[*An Introduction to Metaphysics*, translated by Hulme, London, 1913].

BERNARD (CLAUDE). *Leçons de physiologie experimentale appliquée à la médecine faites au Collège de France*, Paris, 1855.
(Theory of invention in the natural sciences) *Introduction a la méthode experimentale*, Paris, 1850.
[*An Introduction to Experimental Medicine*, translated by Greene, New York, 1927.]

BERTHELOT (MARCELLIN). *Science et philosophie*, Paris, 1886.
On the experimental method.

BERTRAND (J.). *Eloges académiques*, Paris, 1890.
A word on the character and origin of the principal inventions.

BINET. *Psychologie du raisonnement*, Paris, 1896.
The rôle of the imagination in reasoning.
[*The Psychology of Reasoning, based on Experimental Researches in Hypnotism*, translated by Whyte, London, 1899.]

BIOT AND ARAGO. *Recueil d'observations géodésiques, astronomiques, et physiques*, Paris, 1821.
Remarks on physical inventions.

BIRAN (MAINE DE). *Sa vie et ses pensées*, by Naville ; Paris, 1857.
Mémoire sur les perceptions obscures, Paris, 1920.
    Analyses of the various forms of the unconscious in
    perception.
    [*The Influence of Habit on the Faculty of Thinking*, with
    Introduction by G. Boas.]
BOAS. *La défense psychique*, Paris, 1924.
    Quoted apropos of the automatic unconscious.
BOUCAUD. *Esquisse de l'ordre universel*, Paris, 1925.
    Science is presented as a revelation of universal order.
BOUGLE. *Leçons de sociologie sur l'évolution des valeurs*, Paris, 1922.
    Discovery there appears as a personal act.
BOUILLET. *Dictionnaire universel des lettres, des sciences, et des arts*,
    Paris, 1896.
    On inventions in the physical sciences.
BOURDEAU. *L'histoire et les historiens*, Paris, 1888.
    On the rôle of the imagination history.
BOUTY. *La vérité scientifique, sa poursuite*, Paris, 1908.
    On the points of departure of inventions.
BOYER (M. J.). Article in the *Echo de Paris*, 1st March, 1925.
    On Sauria, the inventor of matches.
BROUSSE. *Interférences*, Paris, 1923.
    Quoted to show the analogy between inventions and
    interferences.
CARO (E.). *Philosophie et philosophes*, Paris, 1888.
    On intuition in invention.
CARRA DE VAUX (BARON). *Leibniz* in the collection *Philosophes et
    penseurs*, Paris, 1900.
CAUSTIER (E.). *Sciences naturelles*, Paris, 1923.
    On the spinal cord and unconscious acts.
CHEVALIER (J.). *Descartes*, Paris, 1920.
    Detailed account of his two dreams.
COLSENET. *La vie inconsciente de l'esprit*, Paris, 1880.
    Utilized in setting forth the various forms of unconscious
    activity.
COMTE (AUGUSTE). *Essai sur la philosophie des mathématiques*, Paris,
    1879.
    On order in mathematics.
    Cours de philosophie positive, Paris, 1830, vol. i, 3rd lesson.
    On Experience in Mathematics.
    [*The Positive Philosophy of Auguste Comte*, translated and
    condensed by Martineau, introduction by Frederick Harrison.
    London, 1852.
    The Fundamental Principles of Positive Philosophy, being the
    first two chapters of the *Cours de philosophie positive*, translated
    by Descours and Jones, with Preface by Beesly, London, 1905.]
CROISET (MAURICE). *Eloge de M. Rousselot prononcé à ses obsèques*,
    18th December, 1924.
    On the invention of experimental phonetics.
COURNOT (AUGUSTINE). *Traité de l'enchaînement des idées fonda-
    mentales dans les sciences et dans l'histoire*, Paris, 1911.
    Profound views on the value of historical data in science.
COURSAT. *Vie et travaux des savants modernes*, Paris, 1923.
    Consulted concerning mathematicians.
DARWIN (CHARLES). *On the Origin of Species by means of Natural
    Selection*, London, 1859.
    On the unconscious in biological inventions. *Life and Letters*,
    edited by his son, Francis Darwin. On the origins of the doctrine
    of descent.

DASTRES (A.). In *Revue des du ex mondes*, 1st April, 1900, p. 690.
On the representative element in sensation.
DE LAUNAY (LOUIS). *Le Grand Ampère d'après des documents inédits*, Paris, 1925.
Feeling and the unconscious in Ampère's inventions.
DELVAILLE (JULES). *La vie sociale et l'éducation*, Paris, 1907.
The rôle of doubt and the spirit of inquiry in intellectual education.
DESCARTES (RENE). *Principia philosophica*, Amsterdam, 1652.
On the fundamental ideas of his system.
[*Philosophical Works*, translated by Haldane and Ross, Cambridge, 1911.]
DESDOUITS. *Philosophie de l'inconscient*, Paris, 1852.
Considerable restriction of the domain of the unconscious.
Dictionnaire de l'Academie francaise, concerning the various uses of the words " invention " and " discovery ".
DUMONT. *Théorie scientifique de la sensiblité*, Paris, 1875.
DUTENS. *Recherches sur l'origine des découvertes attribuées aux modernes*, Paris, 1796.
Many recent discoveries have been foreshadowed in the past.
DWELSHAUVERS (G.). *L'inconscient*, Paris, 1916.
The various forms of the unconscious, *Les mécanismes subconscients*, Paris, 1925.
Used especially in the study of the automatic unconscious.
Etudes, 62nd year, No. 22, vol. 185, p. 423, article on the Unconscious.
EYMIEU (ANTONIN). *Le gouvernement de soi-même*, vol. i. *Les grandes lois*, Paris, 1905.
On the idea constantly associated with feeling.
FERRAZ. *La psychologie de Saint Augustin*, Paris, 1865.
The unconscious of memory according to St. Augustine.
FONSEGRIVE (G.). *François Bacon*, Paris, 1893.
The Scientific work of Bacon ; invention in Science.
FORTIS (LE COMTE DE). *Etude historique de Jacquard*, Paris, 1840.
Jacquard, inventor of the pattern loom.
GAUSS. Letter of the 3rd September, 1805, quoted in the *Revue des Questions scientifiques*, Brussels, October, 1884.
In connection with the unconscious in mathematical invention.
GELEY (DR.). *De l'inconscient au conscient*, Paris.
On the nature of the distant unconscious.
GERMAIN (SOPHIE). *Ouvres philosophiques*, Paris, 1878.
On the unconscious in imagination.
GOBLOT (EDMOND). " Sur l'induction mathématique," article in the *Revue philosophique*, 7th April, 1914 ; *Le système des sciences*, Paris, 1922.
The author explains how he discovered the theory of constructive deduction.
GODFERNAUX. *Le sentiment et la pensée et leurs principales applications psychologiques*, Paris, 1894.
On the co-operation of feeling and idea.
GOURMONT (REMY DE). *La création subconsciente*, Paris, 1900.
GRASSET (DR.). *Introduction physiologique à la philosophie*, Paris, 1908 ; *le psychisme inférieur, étude de physio-pathologie clinique des centres nerveux*.
On the unconscious explained by physiology ; the theory of the polygon.
GRATACAP. *Thèse sur la mémoire*, Paris.
Quoted by Colsenet regarding the unconscious in recollection.

HAMILTON (SIR W.). *Lectures on Metaphysics and Logic*, edited by Mansel and Veitch, Edinburgh and London, 1877.
Quoted concerning unconscious acts and states.

HART (ROBERT). " Reminiscences of James Watt," *Transactions of the Glasgow Archeological Society*, 1859.

HARTMAN. *Philosophy of the Unconscious*, translated by William Chatterton Coupland, new edition, London, 1931.

HELMHOLTZ. *Handbuch der physiologischen Optik*, 3rd edition, Hamburg and Leipzig, 1910.
Quoted concerning optical illusions *On the Sensations of Tone as a Physiological Basis for the Theory of Music*, translated by Ellis, 2nd English edition, London, 1885.
The unconscious in the formation of harmonics.

HANNEQUIN. *Étude d'histoire des sciences et d'histoire de la philosophie*, Paris, 1908.
On unity in science and in philosophy.

HERBART. *Psychologie als Wissenschaft* (Introduction).

HERBERT (DR.). *Auto-suggestion*.
On the æsthetic unconscious.

HOEFER. *Histoire de l'astronomie*, Paris, 1873.
On invention in the physical sciences.
Imprimerie (Histoire de l'), Paris, 1840.
Containing Gutenberg's letters concerning his invention.

JANET (PIERRE). *Les médications psychologiques*, Paris, 1919.
Psychological Healing, translated by E. and C. Paul, London and New York, 1925.
On the automatic unconscious.

JASTROW. *The Subconscious*, London, Boston, and New York, 1906.
On the simultaneous disappearance of consciousness and attention.

JESSEN. *Versuch einer wissenschaftlichen Begründung der Psychologie*, Berlin, 1855.
Quoted by Hartmann concerning the unconscious in the change of opinion.

JOANNE (ADOLPHE). *Itineraire de la Savoie*, Paris.
Quoted with reference to perforating machines.

JOLY (H.). *L'imagination*, Paris, 1877.
Rôle and importance of the imagination in intellectual operations.

JOYAU. *De l'invention dans les lettres, dans les sciences, dans les arts et dans la pratique de la vertu*, Paris, 1879.
The author sees in the creative imagination the source of all inventions.

KANT. *Anthropologie in pragmatischer Hinsicht abgefasst*, Königsberg, 1798.
Quoted with reference to unconscious representations.

LAHR (CH.). *Cours de philosophie*, Paris, 1926, 25th edition.
Exact definition of the sense of the world " subconscious ".

LAISANT. *La mathématique*, Paris, 1878.
Part played by the unconscious in the formation of mathematical concepts.

LALANDE. *Lectures sur la philosophie des sciences*, chap. iii.
On experience in mathematics.

LAPLACE. *Essai philosophique sur les probabilités*, Paris, 1840.
A Philosophical Essay on Probabilities, translated by Truscott and Emery, New York, 1902.
Exposition du système du monde, Paris.
On the progressive formation of his cosmic hypothesis.

LAROUSSE. *Dicti-universel*, vol. ix.
Quoted with reference to the meaning of the word invention.

BIBLIOGRAPHY 331

BIBLIOGRAPHY 331

LASBAX (EMILE). *Le problème du mal*, Paris, 1919.
LAUNAY (LOUIS DE). *Le grand Ampère d'après des documents inédits*, Paris, 1925.
Remarkable examples of inventions produced by the phenomena of sensibility, sometimes conscious, sometimes unconscious.
LE BON (GUSTAVE). *La vie des vérités*, Paris, 1914.
The author expounds his theory of residues, the basis of inventions.
LE DANTEC. *Le chaos et l'harmonie universelle*, Paris, 1911.
Critical exposition of the laws of chance.
LEIBNIZ. *New Essays concerning Human Understanding*, translated by Langley, 2nd edition, London and Chicago, 1916.
Principes de la nature et de la grâce fondés en raison, Paris, 1865.
The unconscious considered in memory.
LENOBLE. Article in *l'Enseignement chrétien*, January, 1926, pp. 4, 5.
On the rôle of the imagination in the moral sciences.
LE PLAY. *La réforme sociale*, Tours, 1887.
On invention in the social sciences, a remarkable case of progressive hypothesis.
LE ROY. " La logique de l'invention " in the *Revue de métaphysique et de morale*, 1905.
On the rôle of action in thought.
LITTRÉ. *Dictionnaire de la langue française*, vol. ii.
On the meaning of the words, " discovery " and " invention ".
LORIDAN. *Nos savants*, Tours, 1897.
MAILLET (G.). " Une crise mystique chez Descartes," in the *Revue de métaphysique*, July, 1916.
Regarding the three dreams of Descartes reported by Chevalier.
MAISTRE (J. DE). *Soirées de Saint-Petersbourg*, i, xe entretien.
On intuition in men of genius.
MAUDSLEY. *The Physiology and Pathology of the Mind*, London, 1867, 1876, 1879.
Quoted with reference to the unconscious.
MILL (JOHN STUART). *An Examination of Sir William Hamilton's Philosophy*, London, 1865.
On the unconscious in recollection.
MONGE (G.). *Geometric descriptive*, Paris, 1891.
The unconscious considered in mathematical invention.
MUNIER. *Vers la Beauté eternelle*, Paris, 1912.
On inventions in general, a revelation of universal order.
NAVILLE (ERNEST). *La logique de l'hypothèse*, Paris, 1880.
On the genesis and value of hypotheses.
NEWTON. *The Method of Fluxions and Infinite Series*, translated by Colson from the unpublished Latin original. London, 1736.
The origin of the infinitesimal calculus.
PALIARD. *Le raison selon Maine de Biran*, Paris, 1925.
The rôle of sensibility in intelligence.
Intuition et reflexion. Esquisse d'une dialectique de la connaissance, Paris, 1925.
The author shows the co-penetration of intuitive and deductive logic.
PASCAL (BLAISE). *Traité de l'équilibre des liqueurs et de la pesanteur*, Paris, 1663.
Consulted regarding discoveries relating to atmospheric pressure.
Pensées, vii.
On inventions in general.

PASTEUR (LOUIS). *Quelques réflexions sur la science en France*, Paris, 1871.
On the development of laboratories which are too little supported by the State.

PAULHAN. *L'activité mentale et les éléments de l'esprit*, Paris, 1889.
On the unconscious in judgment.
Les phénomènes affectifs et les lois de leur apparition, Paris, 1887.
On the relation between representative and emotional phenomena.
La fonction de la mémoire et le souvenir affectif, Paris, 1904.
[*The Laws of Feeling*, translated by Ogden, London, 1930].
Platon, chap. v, pp. 167–73–4.
Opinion regarding the distant unconscious.

PICARD (E.). *Pascal, mathématicien et physicien*, Paris, 1923.
On the rôle of desire in mathematical inventions.

POINCARÉ (HENRI), *Science et méthode*, Paris, 1908.
[*Science and Method*, translated by Maitland, London, 1914.]
Description of the circumstances attending his invention of fuchsian functions.
Bibliographie analytique de ses ecrits, Paris, 1912 ; *Savants et écrivains*, Paris, 1912 ; *Leçons sur les hypothèses cosmogoniques*, Paris, 1913.
Concerning sensibility in science ; Poincaré's opinion is given in the notice of E. Lebon.
Dernières pensées, Paris, 1913.
Science is nothing but a candle burning in the night, but this candle is all.

RIBOT (TH.). *Problèmes de psychologie affective*, Paris, 1910 ; *L'imagination créatrice*, Paris, 1900.
[*Essay on the Creative Imagination*, translated by Baron, London and Chicago, 1906.]
In these two works, Ribot throws into relief the emotional factor in imagination.

RICHET (CH.). *L'homme et l'intelligence*, Paris, 1884.
On psychological automatism.

RIGNANO (EUGENIO). *Psychologie du raisonnement*, Paris, 1920.
[*The Psychology of Reasoning*, translated by Hall, London, 1923.]
The unconscious in the discovery of the author's theory concerning the effective and experimental genesis of all reasoning.
Essai de Synthèse scientifique, Paris, 1912.
On the æsthetic unconscious.

SCHIMDT (OSCAR). *Les sciences naturelles et la philosophie de l'inconscient*, Paris, 1879.
The unconscious in the biological sciences.

SCHOPENHAUER. *The World as Will and Idea*, translated by Haldane and Kemp, London, 1883.
The author's conception of the importance of intuition in science.

SEGOND (JOSEPH). *Intuition et amitié*, Paris, 1919.
On the various forms of intuition.
L'intuition Bergsonienne, Paris, 1912.
L'imagination, étude critique, Paris, 1922.
On the imagination considered as a pure power.
" Le raisonnement et l'activité intentionnelle de l'esprit " in the *Journal de psychologie*, 15th December, 1925.
The imagination in invention.

SEGUIN (MARC). *Dictionnaire universel des Contemporains*, p. 1659.

SEIGNOBOS (CH.). *Introduction aux études historiques*, Paris, 1910.
[— and Langlois, C.V. ; *Introduction to the Study of History*,
translated by Berry, London, 1925].
   On the unconscious synthetic work of the imagination in history.
SOMMER. *Petit Dictionnaire des Synonymes français*, Paris.
   Consulted regarding the precise meaning of invention and
discovery.
SORTAIS (GASTON). *Etudes philosophiques et sociales*, Paris.
   Long quotation relating to Newton.
SOURIAU (PAUL). *La beauté rationelle*, Paris, 1904.
   On the rôle of desire in reasoning.
   Théorie de l'invention, Paris, 1881.
   On chance in invention.
   La rêverie esthétique, Paris, 1906.
   On the relations between the conscious and unconscious.
TANNERY. *Science et philosophie*, Paris, 1912.
   On the part played by reading in invention.
TARDE (G.). *Les lois de l'imitation ; la logique sociale*, Paris, 1895.
   [*Social Laws : an Outline of Sociology*, translated by Warren,
New York, 1899.]
   In these two works, this eminent thinker describes the way
in which he discovered the laws of imitation, and develops very
original views on invention in social science.
THOMAS AQUINAS (SAINT). *Adversus Gentes*.
   On intuition.
THOMAS (FELIX). *Cours de philosophie*, Paris, 1921, 8th edition.
   Quoted regarding the analysis of consciousness.
   La suggestion, son rôle dans l'éducation, Paris, 1919.
   Used in the study of the dynamic unconscious.
THURSTON. *A History of the Growth of the Steam Engine*, London,
1872.
   On the invention of engines, chiefly the condenser and
locomotive.
VALLERY-RADOT. *La vie de Pasteur*, Paris, 1900.
   Much information on the origins of his discoveries.
VALSON (C. A.). *La vie et les travaux d'Ampère*, Lyon, 1886.
   On the rôle of feeling in discovery.
VILLEBOIS. *Revue de métaphysique et de morale*, 1901.
   On the plasticity of reason.
VINCENT (C.). *Théorie de la composition littéraire*, Paris, 1916.
   On invention in literature.
WUNDT. *Principles of Physiological Psychology* translated by Titchener,
London, 1902.
   Feeling considered as confused knowledge.
ZURCHER ET MARGOLLE. *L'énergie morale*, Paris, 1882.
   On psychic force, moral force as compared with force in general.

INDEX